WORKBOOK FOR EVIDENCE-BASED PRACTICE IN ACTION

Comprehensive Strategies, Tools, and Tips From the University of Iowa Hospitals and Clinics

Laura Cullen, DNP, RN, FAAN
Kirsten Hanrahan, DNP, ARNP, CPNP-PC
Michele Farrington, BSN, RN, CPHON
Jennifer DeBerg, OT, MLS
Sharon Tucker, PhD, RN, PMHCNS-BC, FAAN
Charmaine Kleiber, PhD, RN, FAAN

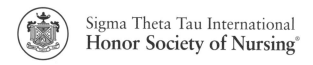

Sigma Theta Tau International
Honor Society of Nursing

The Honor Society of Nursing, Sigma Theta Tau International (STTI) is a nonprofit organization whose mission is advancing world health and celebrating nursing excellence in scholarship, leadership, and service. Founded in 1922, STTI has more than 135,000 active members in over 90 countries and territories. Members include practicing nurses, instructors, researchers, policymakers, entrepreneurs, and others. STTI's 530 chapters are located at more than 700 institutions of higher education throughout Armenia, Australia, Botswana, Brazil, Canada, Colombia, England, Ghana, Hong Kong, Japan, Jordan, Kenya, Lebanon, Malawi, Mexico, the Netherlands, Pakistan, Philippines, Portugal, Singapore, South Africa, South Korea, Swaziland, Sweden, Taiwan, Tanzania, Thailand, the United States, and Wales. Learn more at www.nursingsociety.org

Sigma Theta Tau International
550 West North Street
Indianapolis, IN, USA 46202

To order additional books, buy in bulk, or order for corporate use, contact Nursing Knowledge International at 888. NKI.4YOU (888.654.4968/US and Canada) or +1.317.634.8171 (outside US and Canada).

To request a review copy for course adoption, email solutions@nursingknowledge.org or call 888.NKI.4YOU (888.654.4968/ US and Canada) or +1.317.634.8171 (outside US and Canada).

Suggested citation:

Cullen, L., Hanrahan, K., Farrington, M., DeBerg, J., Tucker, S., & Kleiber, C. (2018). *Workbook for evidence-based practice in action: Comprehensive strategies, tools, and tips from the University of Iowa Hospitals and Clinics.* Indianapolis, IN: Sigma Theta Tau International.

To request author information, or for speaker or other media requests, contact Marketing, Honor Society of Nursing, Sigma Theta Tau International at 888.634.7575 (US and Canada) or +1.317.634.8171 (outside US and Canada).

PRINT ISBN: 9781945157516
PDF ISBN: 9781945157530

First Printing, 2017

Publisher: Dustin Sullivan
Acquisitions Editor: Emily Hatch
Cover Designer: Michael Tanamachi
Page Design & Composition: Tricia Bronkella

Principal Book Editor: Carla Hall
Editorial Coordinator: Paula Jeffers
Proofreader: Todd Lothery
Illustrator: Laura Robbins

About the Authors

LAURA CULLEN, DNP, RN, FAAN

Laura Cullen is an Evidence-Based Practice Scientist at the University of Iowa (UI) Hospitals and Clinics. Cullen is known for her innovative educational programs and for supporting adoption of evidence-based practice (EBP) by point-of-care clinicians and teams. Her work has led to the adoption of innovative practices; improved patient safety; improved patient, family, and clinician satisfaction; reduced hospital length of stay and costs; and transformation of many organizations' infrastructures to support EBP. She has numerous publications and national and international presentations and has received multiple awards for her work. Cullen is Adjunct Faculty at the UI College of Nursing and has served as the U.S. representative on an international panel for the Honor Society of Nursing, Sigma Theta Tau International. Cullen co-authors a regular EBP column in the *Journal of PeriAnesthesia Nursing*, is a member of the editorial board of the *American Journal of Nursing*, and participates on the grant review panel for the DAISY Foundation™. She is a Fellow in the American Academy of Nursing and has been named one of Iowa's 100 Great Nurses.

KIRSTEN HANRAHAN, DNP, ARNP, CPNP-PC

Kirsten Hanrahan is the Interim Director of Nursing Research, Evidence-Based Practice, and Quality at the UI Hospitals and Clinics and a Pediatric Nurse Practitioner transitioning neonatal intensive care unit infants to home from the UI Stead Family Children's Hospital. She is Adjunct Faculty at the UI College of Nursing and is well-versed in EBP and clinical research. Her research interests include pediatric IV management and pain. She has consulted for a National Institutes of Health multi-site study and is co-founder of the Distraction in Action© tool that helps parents learn to be a distraction coach for their child during medical procedures. She is currently the principal investigator for studies related to pediatric intensive care unit pain management, parent distraction for procedural pain, and evaluation of a children's hospital healing environment. Hanrahan has authored evidence-based guidelines and implemented multiple EBP changes in the clinical setting. She has numerous publications and national and international presentations and has been named one of Iowa's 100 Great Nurses.

MICHELE FARRINGTON, BSN, RN, CPHON

Michele Farrington is a Clinical Healthcare Research Associate at the UI Hospitals and Clinics and is certified in pediatric hematology oncology nursing. She serves as a study coordinator and EBP mentor. Previously, she served as a staff nurse in pediatrics and has tremendous experience and expertise in pediatric oncology and EBP, leading or co-leading initiatives since 2003. Her work has been awarded extramural funding, validating the strength of the projects and impact on nursing care. Moreover, she has numerous publications related to EBP projects and has given multiple local, national, and international presentations. Farrington is *ORL – Head and Neck Nursing* Media Review Column Department Editor; AAO-HNSF Guideline Task Force member; Chair of the SOHN Nursing Practice and Research Committee; SOHN National Education Committee member; SOHN Congress Planning Committee member (2016–2019); *EBP to Go®: Accelerating Evidence-Based Practice* Series Editor; and she is actively involved in multiple professional organizations. She is a past recipient of the Nursing Excellence in Clinical Education Award, 100 Great Iowa Nurses Award, and ENT-NF Literary Awards.

JENNIFER DEBERG, OT, MLS

Jennifer DeBerg is a User Services Librarian at the Hardin Library for the Health Sciences at the UI Libraries. She provides information management instruction and services to clinicians, students, faculty, and staff from various health science disciplines. She is Adjunct Lecturer with the UI College of Nursing, where she collaborates with faculty in undergraduate and graduate courses pertaining to research and EBP. Because of previous experience as an occupational therapist, she has a passion for providing support to clinicians related to EBP and quality care. DeBerg is active in several professional organizations, has been a presenter at numerous regional and national conferences, and is a regular contributor to articles published in both library and health sciences journals.

SHARON TUCKER, PHD, RN, PMHCNS-BC, FAAN

Sharon Tucker is the Grayce Sills Endowed Professor in Psychiatric-Mental Health Nursing and Director of the Translational Research Core of the new Helene Fuld Health Trust National Institute for Evidence-Based Practice in the College of Nursing at The Ohio State University (OSU). She assumed this position in 2017 after serving 6 years as the Director of Nursing Research, Evidence-Based Practice, and Quality at the UI Hospitals and Clinics and held a joint appointment at the UI College of Nursing. Tucker's research program relates to understanding and motivating human behaviors through interventions that promote health and reduce health risks, with a particular focus on working mothers and their children. She brings this behavioral expertise to the adoption and translation of evidence-based nursing practices among clinicians. Tucker has extensive clinical, teaching, and research experiences in mental and behavioral health. Through her research, she partners with colleagues from across OSU, UI,

Mayo Clinic, Iowa State University, and Johns Hopkins University. She has extramural funding and support, has published extensively, and actively participates in parent and child wellness initiatives at the local, state, and national levels.

CHARMAINE KLEIBER, PHD, RN, FAAN

Charmaine Kleiber is an Associate Research Scientist at the UI Hospitals and Clinics and Associate Professor Emeritus at the UI College of Nursing. Kleiber's clinical career focused on pediatrics and intensive care. Her research focus is the management of children's pain, especially during medical procedures. Kleiber is co-founder of the Distraction in Action© tool that helps parents learn to be a distraction coach for their child during medical procedures. While on faculty at the UI College of Nursing, Kleiber developed and taught undergraduate and graduate courses for nurses on the conduct of research and EBP. She has been honored by the American Academy of Nursing as an "Edgerunner" for innovative pain management research and by the Midwest Nursing Research Society Pain and Symptom Management Research Interest Groups for "Advancing the Science." She also had a key role in the development and publication of the original Iowa Model and both published revisions.

The Iowa Model Revised: Evidence-Based Practice to Promote Excellence in Health Care

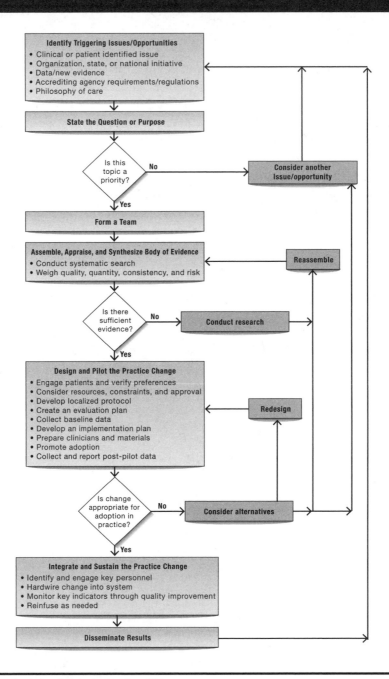

©University of Iowa Hospitals and Clinics, Revised June 2015
To request permission to use or reproduce, go to http://www.uihealthcare.org/nursing-research-and-evidence-based-practice

Iowa Model Collaborative. (2017). Iowa Model of Evidence-Based Practice: Revisions and validation. *Worldviews on Evidence-Based Nursing, 14*(3), 175–182. doi:10.1111/wvh.12223

Overview

Welcome to the companion workbook to *Evidence-Based Practice in Action: Comprehensive Strategies, Tools, and Tips From the University of Iowa Hospitals and Clinics* (Cullen et al., 2018). This workbook provides a description for how to bring evidence-based practice (EBP) improvements into clinical practice. Tools are organized using the Iowa Model Revised: Evidence-Based Practice to Promote Excellence in Health Care© (Iowa Model Collaborative, 2017). There are a variety of models used for EBP. Because EBP process models have similar overarching steps and use the same basic problem-solving process, these tools will be useful regardless of the EBP model.

This workbook was created to provide direct and easy access to EBP tools for busy clinicians. In the pages that follow, you will be given a brief introduction to each chapter along with the tools included to address that step in the EBP process. Refer to *Evidence-Based Practice in Action* for more detailed descriptions, tips, examples, strategies, and additional resources for comprehensive guidance focusing on each component of the EBP process.

Chapter 1: Identify Triggering Issues/Opportunities

EBP begins when clinicians identify practice issues, challenges, or desired changes in outcome metrics. In the Iowa Model, an issue or "trigger" is identified from a clinical problem, organizational initiative, or new knowledge. The purpose of EBP is to solve the problem or compare new knowledge to current practice. Identification of triggers may originate from any member of the healthcare team but often comes from clinicians questioning current practice.

Tool 1.1: Potential EBP Topics

Chapter 2: State the Question or Purpose

This is a new formal step in the Iowa Model. The following tools help when formulating actionable questions using the PICO (P = patient/problem/population, I = intervention, C = comparison, O = outcome) framework (Schardt, Adams, Owens, Keitz, & Fontelo, 2007). The PICO components are used to develop the project's purpose statement, which helps set boundaries around the project work.

Tool 2.1: PICO Concepts for Developing a Purpose Statement
Tool 2.2: PICO Elements for a Purpose Statement and Evidence Search

Chapter 3: Is This Topic a Priority?

Identification of priority topics is essential as not every clinical question can be addressed through the EBP process. Higher priority may be given to topics that address high volume, high risk, or high cost issues; those that are closely aligned with the institution's strategic plan; or other institutional or market forces (e.g., patient or clinician safety, changing reimbursement). If the topic is not an organizational priority, clinicians may want to consider a different focus, different project outcomes, or other opportunities for improving practice. This and similar feedback loops within the Iowa Model highlight that the work is not linear, so feedback loops are suggested.

Tool 3.1: Determining if Topic Is a Priority

Tool 3.2: Linking EBP Topic With Organizational Priorities

Tool 3.3: EBP Topic Selection

Chapter 4: Form a Team

Once there is commitment to address the topic, an EBP team should be formed to develop, implement, and evaluate the practice change. EBP team membership requires several considerations to ensure the correct clinicians are involved and to maximize use of the team members' skills and organizational functions and structures.

Tool 4.1: EBP Project Timeline

Tool 4.2: General Action Plan

Chapter 5: Assemble, Appraise, and Synthesize Body of Evidence

The EBP team selects, critiques, and synthesizes the best available evidence. A comprehensive literature search must be completed before all the available evidence is critically reviewed and synthesized to make a recommendation for practice.

Tool 5.1: Assembling Evidence

Tool 5.2: Record of Search History and Yield by Source

Tool 5.3: Appraisal and Synthesis of Evidence

Tool 5.4: Summary and Synthesis Table

Tool 5.5: AGREE II Instrument

Tool 5.6: Appraise Evidence

Tool 5.7: Systematic Review Appraisal

Tool 5.8: Quantitative Research Appraisal

Tool 5.9: Qualitative Research Appraisal

Tool 5.10: Other Evidence Appraisal

Chapter 6: Is There Sufficient Evidence?

At this point, the entire body of evidence—including research, case studies, quality data, expert opinions, and patient input—is synthesized. During this step, the team determines when the evidence is considered sufficient, or not sufficient, for pilot testing.

Tool 6.1: Determine if There Is Sufficient Evidence

Tool 6.2: Determining Quality Improvement, EBP, or Research

Chapter 7: Design and Pilot the Practice Change

Piloting is an essential step in the EBP process. Outcomes achieved in a controlled research environment may result in different outcomes than those found when EBP is used in a real-world clinical setting. Piloting the EBP change is essential for identifying issues with the intervention, implementation, and potential rollout to multiple clinical areas.

Tool 7.1: Determining a Need for a Policy or Procedure

Chapter 8: Implementation

Implementation is fluid, complex, and highly interactive, and it changes over the course of the pilot period. Multiple implementation strategies are selected and used cumulatively to create a comprehensive plan based on the four phases of implementation: creating awareness and interest, building knowledge and commitment, promoting action and adoption, and pursuing integration and sustainability (Cullen & Adams, 2012).

Tool 8.1: Selecting Implementation Strategies for EBP

Tool 8.2: Collecting Pilot Process Issues

Chapter 9: Evaluation

Evaluation of the pilot must focus on select key indicators related specifically to the practice change and for input to guide implementation. Both process and outcome indicators are collected before and after implementation of the practice change. A few key indicators will be monitored until the improvement is sustained.

Tool 9.1: Selecting Process and Outcome Indicators

Tool 9.2: Developing Topic-Specific Process and Outcome Indicators

Tool 9.3: Audit Form

Tool 9.4: Clinician Questionnaire

Chapter 10: Is Change Appropriate for Adoption in Practice?

This decision point requires the EBP team to either recommend adoption of the practice change or pursue other courses of action.

Tool 10.1: Decision to Adopt an EBP

Tool 10.2: EBP Framework for Making Decisions About Adoption of EBP in Practice

Tool 10.3: Decision to Implement

Chapter 11: Integrate and Sustain the Practice Change

This step promotes integration and sustainability of the practice change over time and prevents regression to previous practice habits. The importance of "hardwiring" the change into the system, tracking evaluative data over time, and planning for periodic reinfusion is emphasized.

Tool 11.1: Action Plan for Sustaining EBP

Tool 11.2: Histograms

Tool 11.3: Run Charts

Tool 11.4: Statistical Process Control Charts

Chapter 12: Disseminate Results

Dissemination of project results is a key step in the EBP process to promote the adoption of EBPs within the larger healthcare community (Sigma Theta Tau International 2005–2007 Research and Scholarship Advisory Committee, 2008). Sharing project reports within and outside the organization through presentation and publication supports the growth of an EBP culture in the organization, expands nursing knowledge, and encourages EBP updates in other settings.

Tool 12.1: Creating an EBP Poster

Tool 12.2: Institutional Review Board Considerations

Tool 12.3: EBP Abstract Template

Tool 12.4: Preparing an EBP Presentation

Tool 12.5: Planning for an EBP Publication

References

Cullen, L., & Adams, S. L. (2012). Planning for implementation of evidence-based practice. *Journal of Nursing Administration, 42*(4), 222–230. doi:10.1097/NNA.0b013e31824ccd0a

Iowa Model Collaborative. (2017). Iowa Model of Evidence-Based Practice: Revisions and validation. *Worldviews on Evidence-Based Nursing, 14*(3), 175–182. doi:10.1111/wvn.12223

Schardt, C., Adams, M. B., Owens, T., Keitz, S., & Fontelo, P. (2007). Utilization of the PICO framework to improve searching PubMed for clinical questions. *BMC Medical Informatics and Decision Making, 7*(16), 1–6. doi:10.1186/1472-6947-7-16

Sigma Theta Tau International 2005–2007 Research and Scholarship Advisory Committee. (2008). Sigma Theta Tau International position statement on evidence-based practice. February 2007 summary. *Worldviews on Evidence-Based Nursing, 5*(2), 57–59. doi:10.1111/j.1741-6787.2008.00118.x

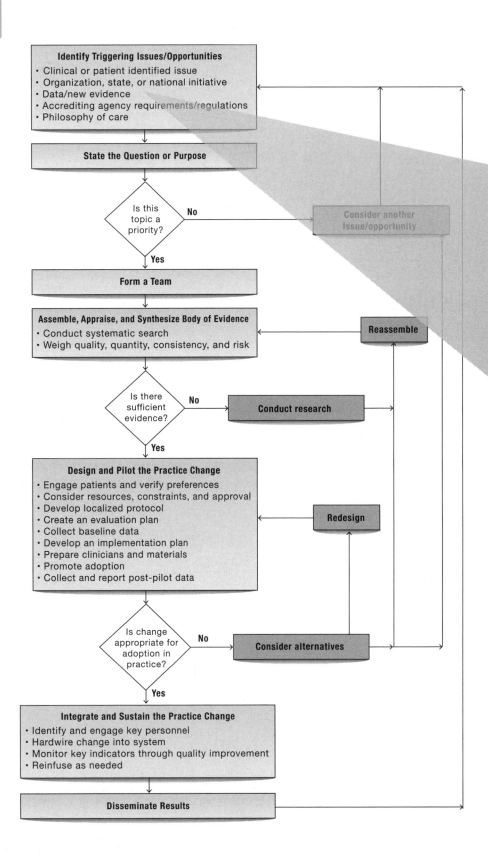

Identify Triggering Issues/Opportunities
- Clinical or patient identified issue
- Organization, state, or national initiative
- Data/new evidence
- Accrediting agency requirements/regulations
- Philosophy of care

State the Question or Purpose

Is this topic a priority?

No → Consider another issue/opportunity

Yes

Form a Team

Assemble, Appraise, and Synthesize Body of Evidence
- Conduct systematic search
- Weigh quality, quantity, consistency, and risk

Reassemble

Is there sufficient evidence?

No → **Conduct research**

Yes

Design and Pilot the Practice Change
- Engage patients and verify preferences
- Consider resources, constraints, and approval
- Develop localized protocol
- Create an evaluation plan
- Collect baseline data
- Develop an implementation plan
- Prepare clinicians and materials
- Promote adoption
- Collect and report post-pilot data

Redesign

Is change appropriate for adoption in practice?

No → **Consider alternatives**

Yes

Integrate and Sustain the Practice Change
- Identify and engage key personnel
- Hardwire change into system
- Monitor key indicators through quality improvement
- Reinfuse as needed

Disseminate Results

IDENTIFY TRIGGERING ISSUES/OPPORTUNITIES

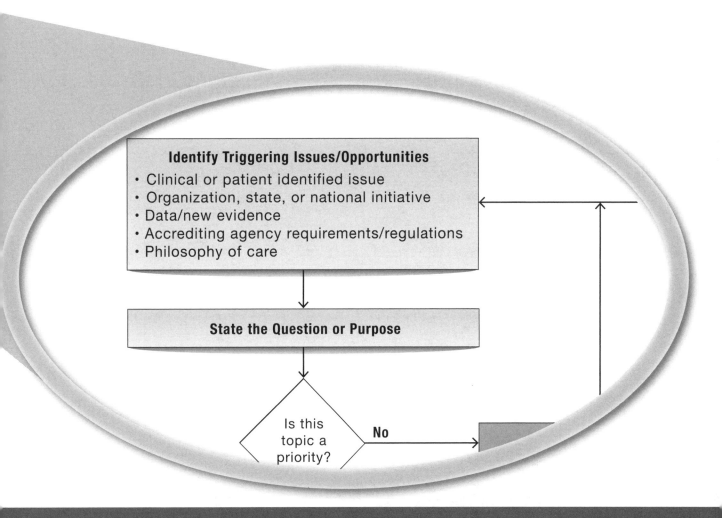

Identify Triggering Issues/Opportunities
- Clinical or patient identified issue
- Organization, state, or national initiative
- Data/new evidence
- Accrediting agency requirements/regulations
- Philosophy of care

State the Question or Purpose

Is this topic a priority?

No

"If I have ever made any valuable discoveries, it has been owing more to patient attention than to any other talent."

–Isaac Newton

EBP begins when clinicians identify practice issues, challenges, or desired changes in outcome metrics. In the Iowa Model, an issue or "trigger" is identified from a clinical problem, organizational initiative, or new knowledge. The purpose of EBP is to solve the problem or compare new knowledge to current practice. Identification of triggers may originate from any member of the healthcare team but often comes from clinicians questioning current practice.

TOOL NAME	PAGE

Tool 1.1   Potential EBP Topics

INSTRUCTIONS: Read the questions below and record your responses. Skip questions that do not apply and proceed to the next question. Take these ideas to a leader and discuss each to identify a topic of interest.

Clinical or Patient Identified Issue

What are the procedures you spend a lot of time doing or do frequently?

getting vitals & doing H-T assessment

What questions are patients and families asking?

how do we get them to eat? Skin is worsening

Who are the high volume patients?

Cancer

Who are the patients with highest risk for a poor outcome?

Head & Neck pts

Organization, State, or National Initiative

Is there a new practice in the organization (e.g., policy) that needs to be implemented?

Are there benchmarks for new practices that you would like to try?

Do you know of a new protocol (i.e., policy, procedure, or standard) that could improve practice?

What is interesting to you among the current organizational initiatives?

Are there clinical practices that can be linked to the strategic plan?

Where could cost savings be achieved?

Data/New Evidence

Are there quality data that you want to improve?

What did you learn at the last conference or program you attended?

When you read journals, which articles are you drawn toward first?

Is your professional organization publishing on topics of interest (e.g., guidelines, position statements)?

Are you aware of research findings that might apply to your practice?

Accrediting Agency Requirements/Regulations

Which regulatory standards would you be interested in addressing through a practice improvement?

What are National Patient Safety Goals for improving quality care?

Are there anticipated or new reimbursement structures (e.g., revisions to value-based purchasing)?

Philosophy of Care

Where is care missing in daily practice (e.g., holistic or comfort interventions)?

What common patient/family experiences could be improved?

Has patient/family shared their experience in a way you had not anticipated?

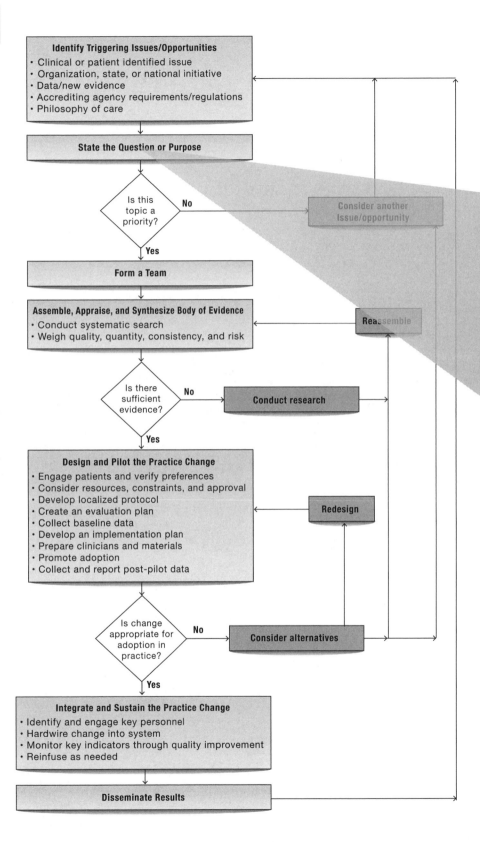

Identify Triggering Issues/Opportunities
- Clinical or patient identified issue
- Organization, state, or national initiative
- Data/new evidence
- Accrediting agency requirements/regulations
- Philosophy of care

State the Question or Purpose

Is this topic a priority?

No → Consider another issue/opportunity

Yes

Form a Team

Assemble, Appraise, and Synthesize Body of Evidence
- Conduct systematic search
- Weigh quality, quantity, consistency, and risk

Reassemble

Is there sufficient evidence?

No → **Conduct research**

Yes

Design and Pilot the Practice Change
- Engage patients and verify preferences
- Consider resources, constraints, and approval
- Develop localized protocol
- Create an evaluation plan
- Collect baseline data
- Develop an implementation plan
- Prepare clinicians and materials
- Promote adoption
- Collect and report post-pilot data

Redesign

Is change appropriate for adoption in practice?

No → **Consider alternatives**

Yes

Integrate and Sustain the Practice Change
- Identify and engage key personnel
- Hardwire change into system
- Monitor key indicators through quality improvement
- Reinfuse as needed

Disseminate Results

STATE THE QUESTION OR PURPOSE

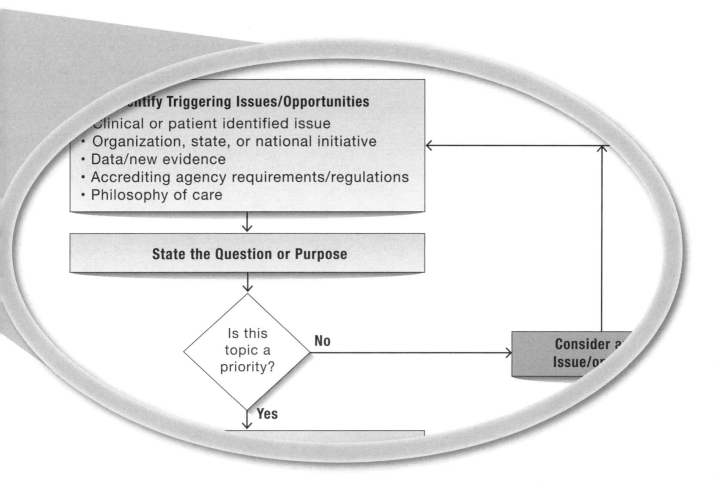

"You can tell whether a man is clever by his answers. You can tell whether a man is wise by his questions."

–Naguib Mahfouz

This is a new formal step in the Iowa Model. The following tools help when formulating actionable questions using the PICO (P = patient/problem/population, I = intervention, C = comparison, O = outcome) framework (Schardt, Adams, Owens, Keitz, & Fontelo, 2007). The PICO components are used to develop the project's purpose statement, which helps set boundaries around the project work.

Mahli Hartmann

Tool 2.1   PICO Concepts for Developing a Purpose Statement

INSTRUCTIONS: Use this worksheet to explore concepts of interest for your EBP work. Organize using the PICO elements. Begin by identifying a goal or outcome first. Identify potential interventions last; interventions may evolve after reading the evidence. Use all PICO elements to write a purpose statement in one to two sentences. Use PICO elements to identify potential keywords related to the purpose statement.

Patient Population

Head & Neck Cancer Patients

Clinical Problem or Condition

Skin breakdown from radiation burns

Pilot Area

Radiation Oncology Clinic

Interventions

Good, balanced & adequate nutrition before & during radiation

Comparison

Poor nutrition or undernutrition during radiation

Anticipated Outcomes

Less skin breakdown & severity

EBP Purpose Statement

Are head & neck cancer patients who have adequate nutrition before & during radiation treatments at decreased risk for skin breakdown & severity of radiation burns as compared with poor or inadequate nutrition?

Keywords or Concepts for Identifying and Organizing Literature

Radiation, Head & neck cancer, skin integrity, health quality, nutrition

Tool 2.2   PICO Elements for a Purpose Statement and Evidence Search

INSTRUCTIONS: Use this worksheet to develop a purpose statement or question. Describe each PICO element addressing the topic of interest. Identify the outcome before considering interventions; interventions may evolve after reading the evidence. Write a purpose statement and determine the kind of question. Use Table 2.1 to identify study designs most likely to answer this question. List related concepts, inclusion and exclusion criteria, and keywords or concepts for organizing evidence.

Step 1: Define elements or clinical question using PICO:

P = Patients or population to target: _Head & Neck Cancer patients_

    Problem or condition to address: _Skin breakdown & radiation burns_

    Pilot area (e.g., unit/clinic): _Rad Onc clinic_

I = Intervention (assessment or treatment): _Good adequate nutrition before & during radiation treatments_

C = Comparison: _Poor nutrition cancer patients_

O = Outcomes: _less skin breakdown, less severe radiation burns, increased healing time_

T = Time frame (optional): _3-6 wks_

Step 2: Purpose statement: _Will good nutrition of head & neck cancer patients improve skin condition and shorten healing time from radiation treatments as compared to those with poor nutrition._

Step 3: Determine what your question is about (circle one):

Therapy   Diagnosis   Etiology   (Prognosis)   Meaning

Step 4: Identify study types that best address your question (circle one or more):

(Experimental studies)   (Observational studies)   Qualitative studies

(Systematic review or meta-analysis)   (Case reports)   Other

Step 5: List the <u>main terms and synonyms</u> for your <u>purpose statement</u>. Typical number of concepts per question is two to three.

Concept 1: Healing time	Concept 2: Good Nutrition	Concept 3: Skin breakdown

- Skin integrity intact
- Improved skin
	- Adequate fluids &
	  Proteins
	  - Balanced nutrition
		- 1st - 3rd degree radiation
		  burns
		- Weeping, erythema

Step 6: List inclusion and exclusion criteria: _exclude those c̄ radiation less than 2wks, include all head & neck CA that receive radiation_

Step 7: Keywords or concepts for organizing literature: _Radiation, head & neck, impaired skin integrity, radiation burn, slowed wound healing._

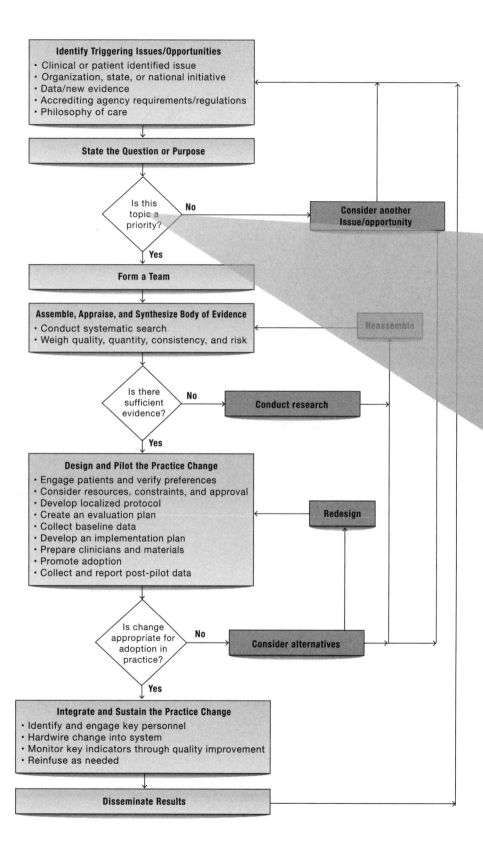

Identify Triggering Issues/Opportunities
- Clinical or patient identified issue
- Organization, state, or national initiative
- Data/new evidence
- Accrediting agency requirements/regulations
- Philosophy of care

State the Question or Purpose

Is this topic a priority?

No → **Consider another Issue/opportunity**

Yes

Form a Team

Assemble, Appraise, and Synthesize Body of Evidence
- Conduct systematic search
- Weigh quality, quantity, consistency, and risk

Reassemble

Is there sufficient evidence?

No → **Conduct research**

Yes

Design and Pilot the Practice Change
- Engage patients and verify preferences
- Consider resources, constraints, and approval
- Develop localized protocol
- Create an evaluation plan
- Collect baseline data
- Develop an implementation plan
- Prepare clinicians and materials
- Promote adoption
- Collect and report post-pilot data

Redesign

Is change appropriate for adoption in practice?

No → **Consider alternatives**

Yes

Integrate and Sustain the Practice Change
- Identify and engage key personnel
- Hardwire change into system
- Monitor key indicators through quality improvement
- Reinfuse as needed

Disseminate Results

IS THIS TOPIC A PRIORITY?

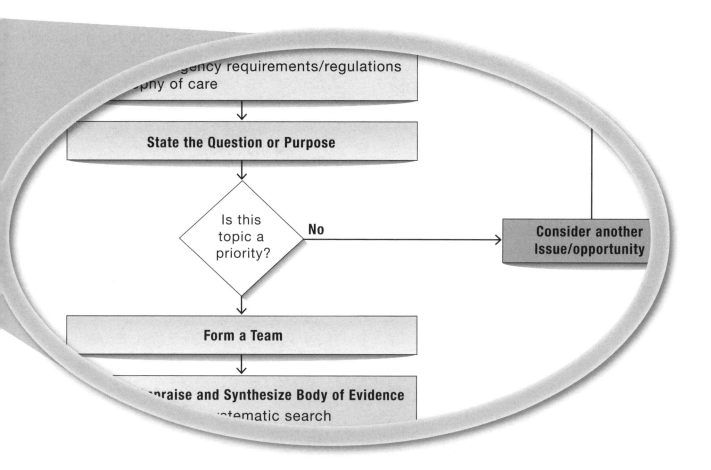

gency requirements/regulations
ephy of care

State the Question or Purpose

Is this
topic a
priority?   **No**   **Consider another
Issue/opportunity**

Form a Team

praise and Synthesize Body of Evidence
atematic search

"Often he who does too much does too little."

–Italian proverb

dentification of priority topics is essential as not every clinical question can be addressed through the EBP process. Higher priority may be given to topics that address high volume, high risk, or high cost issues; those that are closely aligned with the institution's strategic plan; or other institutional or market forces (e.g., patient or clinician safety, changing reimbursement). If the topic is not an organizational priority, clinicians may want to consider a different focus, different project outcomes, or other opportunities for improving practice. This and similar feedback loops within the Iowa Model highlight that the work is not linear, so feedback loops are suggested.

TOOLS

Tool 3.1   Determining if Topic Is a Priority

INSTRUCTIONS: This worksheet is designed to help you determine whether a new clinical or operational question is a priority for your setting or organization. Use it individually, in groups, or as a point for discussion when reviewing the EBP purpose statement.

1. To what extent do you agree that this topic:

		Strongly Agree	Agree	Disagree	Strongly Disagree
a)	Addresses a common or high-priority problem in our practice or setting	1	2	3	4
b)	Is relevant to patients' preferences for care and/or quality of life	1	2	3	4
c)	Has an economic burden associated with it (e.g., readmission, lost work time)	1	2	3	4
d)	Is likely to improve processes or patient outcomes in our practice or setting	1	2	3	4
e)	Would improve safety for our patients, their families, clinicians, or other staff	1	2	3	4
f)	Has new evidence or quality data that identify a need to change	1	2	3	4
g)	Provides an opportunity for innovative practice improvement	1	2	3	4

2. To what extent would this be a priority based on:

		Low			High	Don't Know
a)	Matches organizational or department strategic plan	1	2	3	4	
b)	Matches messages from executives	1	2	3	4	
c)	Is linked to an established core metric	1	2	3	4	
d)	Is part of a new initiative	1	2	3	4	
e)	Is a publicly reported measure	1	2	3	4	
f)	Addresses an accreditation or regulatory standard	1	2	3	4	
g)	Has an established sponsor or is part of a supported training program (e.g., EBP internship, leadership training)	1	2	3	4	

3. Are there any other considerations for determining the priority for this topic?

_____

_____

Tool 3.2 Linking EBP Topic With Organizational Priorities

INSTRUCTIONS: Write the purpose statement at the top. Identify the scope of the problem (e.g., consider patient volume), using data where possible. Identify where the topic and scope of the problem match elements in the next sections. Identify the sponsor or sponsoring program, as an additional indication the topic matches stakeholder priorities.

EBP Purpose Statement or Goal

Scope of the Problem

Organizational Considerations

☐ Links to organization mission/vision/values or initiatives (specify):

☐ Existing data–data source:

☐ Gap analysis or organizational assessment:

Impact for Patient and/or Family

☐ Matches patient preferences:

☐ Impact on quality of life:

☐ Other:

Economic Considerations

☐ Hospital costs (e.g., readmission, length of stay):

☐ Patient and/or family costs (e.g., lost work time):

☐ Resource requirements:

☐ Other:

Established Sponsorship

☐ Sponsor:

☐ Program:

©University of Iowa Hospitals and Clinics, Revised June 2017

Tool 3.3　EBP Topic Selection

INSTRUCTIONS: Identify topics of interest to patients or families, clinicians, or teams. Use more than one sheet if many topics have been identified. Individually review the topics and select a rating; rate each topic using a 0–10 scale (0 = Not at all; 10 = Exceptional). Tally a total score for each topic. Share scores as a group. Discuss the rationale for selecting highest scoring topics. Make a selection as a group.

Review Criteria	Criteria Met/Points	Topic 1	Topic 2	Topic 3
Topic addresses a departmental or organizational priority	0–10			
Priority for the patient population or the unit	0–10			
Topic is an issue that is amenable to being addressed through the EBP process (versus research) and addresses quality or safety	0–10			
Magnitude of the problem for the population (e.g., high risk or high volume)	0–10			
Sufficient evidence available to guide practice	0–10			
Likelihood of improving patient, family, clinician, or fiscal outcomes	0–10			
Sufficient team/interprofessional support or is linked to the work of an existing committee or work group	0–10			
Sufficient resources (e.g., patient health record data, data management for evaluation, reporting, equipment, purchase mailing list, clinical expertise)	0–10			
Other criteria:	0–10			
Rating scale: 0 = Not at all; 10 = Exceptional	Total score(s):			

TOOLS

20

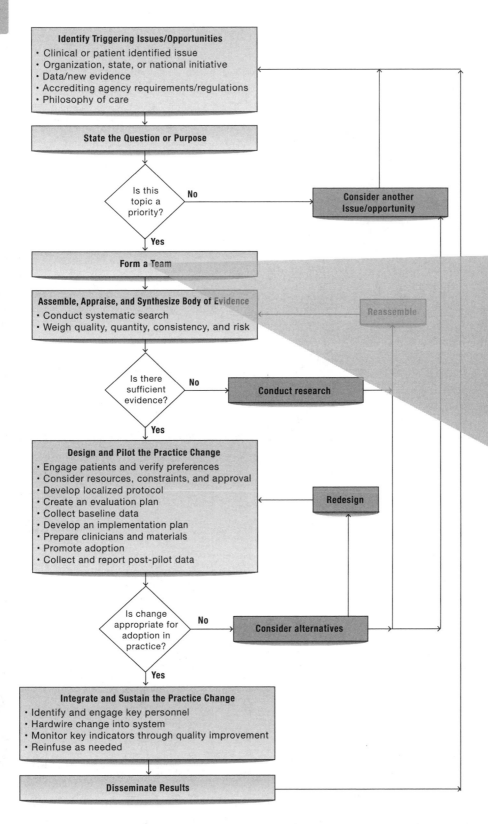

Identify Triggering Issues/Opportunities
- Clinical or patient identified issue
- Organization, state, or national initiative
- Data/new evidence
- Accrediting agency requirements/regulations
- Philosophy of care

State the Question or Purpose

Is this topic a priority?

No — Consider another Issue/opportunity

Yes

Form a Team

Assemble, Appraise, and Synthesize Body of Evidence
- Conduct systematic search
- Weigh quality, quantity, consistency, and risk

Reassemble

Is there sufficient evidence?

No — Conduct research

Yes

Design and Pilot the Practice Change
- Engage patients and verify preferences
- Consider resources, constraints, and approval
- Develop localized protocol
- Create an evaluation plan
- Collect baseline data
- Develop an implementation plan
- Prepare clinicians and materials
- Promote adoption
- Collect and report post-pilot data

Redesign

Is change appropriate for adoption in practice?

No — Consider alternatives

Yes

Integrate and Sustain the Practice Change
- Identify and engage key personnel
- Hardwire change into system
- Monitor key indicators through quality improvement
- Reinfuse as needed

Disseminate Results

FORM A TEAM

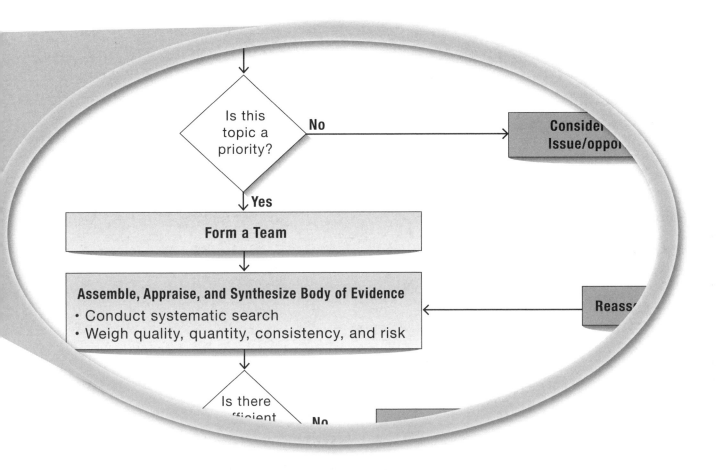

Once there is commitment to address the topic, an EBP team should be formed to develop, implement, and evaluate the practice change. EBP team membership requires several considerations to ensure the correct clinicians are involved and to maximize use of the team members' skills and organizational functions and structures.

Tool 4.1   EBP Project Timeline

INSTRUCTIONS: Insert the month as a header for each numbered column. Review the steps in the process and add any additional steps that would be helpful. Shade boxes for each step that correspond to the anticipated month it will be completed.

Activity	1	2	3	4	5	6	7	8	9	10	11	12	13	14	15	16	17
Define EBP purpose and team																	
Assemble, appraise, and synthesize evidence																	
Design practice change																	
Plan pilot and create resource materials																	
Collect baseline data																	
Prepare change agents																	
Prepare clinicians																	
Implement																	
Evaluate post-pilot																	
Begin project reporting																	
Begin project integration and continue monitoring																	

Go Live ➚

Strategy 1: Implement strategies to create awareness and interest.

Strategy 2: Implement strategies to build knowledge and commitment.

Strategy 3: Implement strategies to promote action and adoption.

Strategy 4: Implement strategies to pursue integration and sustainability.

NOTE: EBP is not a linear process. Strategies often overlap, and time frames may need to be adjusted.

24

TOOLS

Tool 4.2   General Action Plan

INSTRUCTIONS: Identify key steps or objectives from the EBP process model. For each key step, add multiple activities that will be needed to complete that step. For each activity, list a specific person responsible, materials or resources needed, an anticipated timeline for completion, and an evaluative metric indicating successful completion (see Strategy 2-22).

Project director name:

Team:

Project purpose:

Key Step or Objective	Specific Activities to Meet Objective	Person Responsible	Materials or Resources Needed	Timeline	Evaluation				

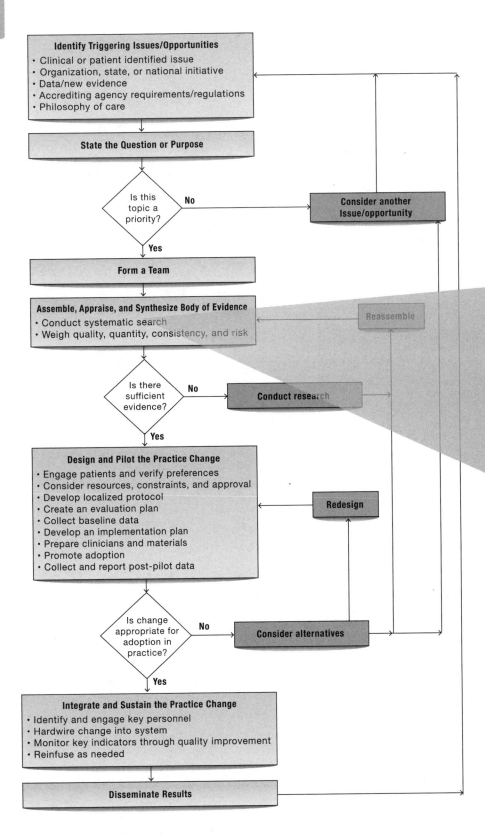

Identify Triggering Issues/Opportunities
- Clinical or patient identified issue
- Organization, state, or national initiative
- Data/new evidence
- Accrediting agency requirements/regulations
- Philosophy of care

State the Question or Purpose

Is this topic a priority?

No → **Consider another Issue/opportunity**

Yes

Form a Team

Assemble, Appraise, and Synthesize Body of Evidence
- Conduct systematic search
- Weigh quality, quantity, consistency, and risk

Reassemble

Is there sufficient evidence?

No → **Conduct research**

Yes

Design and Pilot the Practice Change
- Engage patients and verify preferences
- Consider resources, constraints, and approval
- Develop localized protocol
- Create an evaluation plan
- Collect baseline data
- Develop an implementation plan
- Prepare clinicians and materials
- Promote adoption
- Collect and report post-pilot data

Redesign

Is change appropriate for adoption in practice?

No → **Consider alternatives**

Yes

Integrate and Sustain the Practice Change
- Identify and engage key personnel
- Hardwire change into system
- Monitor key indicators through quality improvement
- Reinfuse as needed

Disseminate Results

ASSEMBLE, APPRAISE, AND SYNTHESIZE BODY OF EVIDENCE

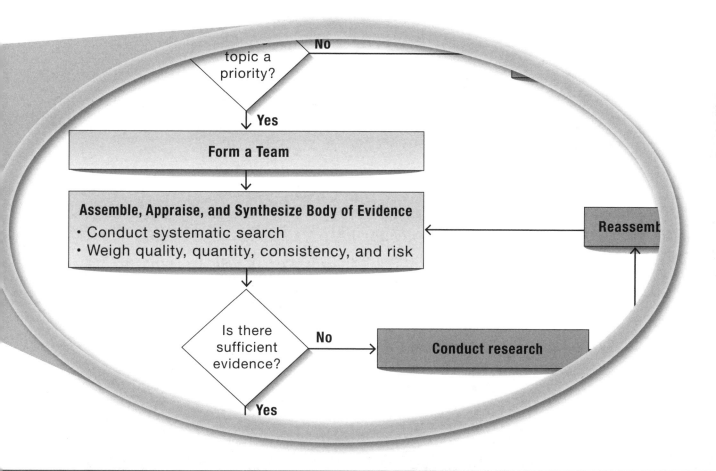

"*The search for truth is in one way hard and in another way easy, for it is evident that no one can master it fully or miss it wholly. But each adds a little to our knowledge of nature, and from all the facts assembled there arises a certain grandeur.*"

–Aristotle

The EBP team selects, critiques, and synthesizes the best available evidence. A comprehensive literature search must be completed before all the available evidence is critically reviewed and synthesized to make a recommendation for practice.

Tool 5.1   Assembling Evidence

INSTRUCTIONS: Review the steps outlined for planning how to assemble the best evidence. Identify dates and times for relevant steps, such as meeting with a health science librarian. Check when steps are completed. Proceed to the next step until each step has been completed.

Date Scheduled	Activity	Done
	Set up meeting with healthcare librarian or use tutorial (such as PubMed) for completing your own database searches. (Online lecture Recording)	☑
	Identify MeSH terms, keywords, and search strategies (e.g., limits) for literature searches based on PICO (Patient population/problem/pilot area, Intervention, Comparison, Outcome) components and purpose statement.	☑
	Complete literature search; save search history and article abstracts; continue updating and recording the searches.	☑
	Locate clinical practice guidelines (if available) first, searching the National Guideline Clearinghouse and other professional organizations.	☑
	Search PubMed, CINAHL, and other large search engines appropriate to the subject or discipline.	☑
	Search the Cochrane Library.	☑
	Search professional organizations' online resources.	☑
	Search other related websites.	☑
	Have at least two reviewers read abstracts to screen articles for relevance and inclusion/exclusion criteria. Where there is a lack of consensus, full articles may be retrieved for further review.	☑
	Retrieve full articles for review. Keep an electronic copy in a reference manager or shared file. Save references in electronic folders by topic, using a standardized format (i.e., first author, subject, year), or provide direct links for easy access by the team.	☑
	Start a reference list using RefWorks, EndNote, or another reference manager, and enter articles as they are retrieved.	☑
	Sort articles according to a) clinical practice guidelines, b) systematic reviews and other synthesis reports, c) research reports, d) theory articles, and e) clinical reviews.	☑
	Read clinical practice guidelines and systematic review articles first to gain understanding of state of practice and science, respectively.	☑
	Read research reports to gain understanding of study design and methods, intervention, variables and measures, relevance to population, and results.	☑
	Read clinical and theoretical articles to gain understanding of theoretical principles and concepts.	☑
	Identify up to 10 key clinical, research, theory, or review articles for the entire team to read.	☑

TOOLS

Tool 5.2   Record of Search History and Yield by Source

INSTRUCTIONS: When using bibliographic databases, save the search history. Include the terms used, how terms were combined, and the yield from each search.

Database	Search or MeSH Term (List)	Approaches for Combining Terms (Boolean Operators AND/OR/NOT)	Limits Used	Yield (Combined Keywords and Numbers of Articles Identified)
National Guideline Clearinghouse (NGC): A public resource for summaries of evidence-based clinical practice guidelines. https://guideline.gov				
The Cochrane Library: The leading resource for systematic reviews in healthcare. http://onlinelibrary.wiley.com/cochranelibrary/search	Radiation & Nutrition	radiation therapy & Nutrition & skin integrity	3	total 13 populated
PubMed: PubMed is composed of more than 26 million citations for biomedical literature from MEDLINE, life science journals, and online books. www.ncbi.nlm.nih.gov/pubmed	Radiation & Skin & Nutrition	radiation & Nutrition & skin flavor	2	→827 populated →20 Nurrured used & citations
CINAHL: CINAHL Plus with full text indexes over 5,000 journals from the fields of nursing and allied health, with indexing back to 1937. https://health.ebsco.com/products/cinahl-plus-with-full-text	radiation & skin & Nutrition	Radiation & Nutrition & skin treatment	4	8 populated
Source: Link:				
Source: Link:				
Source: Link:				
Source: Link:				

Tool 5.3   Appraisal and Synthesis of Evidence

INSTRUCTIONS: Review the steps outlined for planning how to appraise and synthesize the available evidence. Identify dates and times for relevant steps, such as meetings to resolve disagreements about inclusion or exclusion. Check when steps are completed. Proceed to the next step until each step has been completed.

Date Scheduled	Activity	Done
	Read articles once while searching and screening the literature.	☑
	Label each article by design (e.g., systematic review, randomized clinical trial).	☑
	Outline a systematic critique process for thoroughly reviewing evidence once.	☑
	Identify criteria for inclusion/exclusion of evidence based on the quality and relevance to practice.	☑
	Determine how to resolve disagreements.	☑
	Create a resource binder and/or electronic folders to organize materials (i.e., articles, guidelines, synthesis tables, practice recommendations, executive summaries, reference lists).	☑
	Create a summary and synthesis table for articles and guidelines and update as materials are read.	☑
	For a large number of articles, arrange literature within the synthesis table by key concepts that will relate directly to practice recommendations.	☑
	Appraise individual evidence-based guidelines and systematic reviews.	☑
	Appraise research articles.	☑
	Appraise theoretical, clinical, and other types of literature.	☑
	Determine inclusion/exclusion for each piece of evidence based on the quality and relevance to established practice criteria.	☑
	Determine the quality, relevance to practice, risks, and key findings for each article or guideline.	☑
	Resolve disagreements about inclusion/exclusion of evidence.	☑
	Compare, contrast, and synthesize information from articles on the synthesis tables.	☑

TOOLS

Tool 5.4   Summary and Synthesis Table

INSTRUCTIONS: Add a brief description for each article into a row. Include enough citation information to locate the article again later, or use APA format to save time doing this later. Briefly include the key elements found while reading that are relevant to the topic. Include only what is helpful and not a comprehensive list of findings. Include key findings and comment on strengths or weaknesses for each article.

Guidelines, Reviews, and Other Literature

Citation	Critique: Type of Evidence/Limitations	Scope	Relevant Findings	Other
Enteral feeding Methods for nutritional management in pts of H&N cancers	Systematic being tx c Rtx &/or Chemo		Tube feedings improve outcome	randomize control
Author: B. Nugent, S. Lewis, J. O'Sullivan				
Increased skin & Mucosal toxicity Authors: R. Merten, M. Hecht, M. Haderlein, etc.				

Research

Citation	Subjects	Design/ Methods	Outcomes	Relevant Results and Findings	Limitations/ Comments

Supplemental Evidence
(not meeting inclusion criteria but supplementing guideline content and literature review)

Citation	Type/Evidence	Scope	Supplemental Information	Comments/Other

Tool 5.5   AGREE II Instrument

The Appraisal of Guidelines for Research and Evaluation (AGREE©) Instrument evaluates the process of practice guideline development and the quality of reporting. The original AGREE Instrument has been updated and methodologically refined. The AGREE II is now the international tool for the assessment of practice guidelines. The AGREE II, which is both valid and reliable, is composed of 23 items organized into the original six quality domains. Appraisals can be completed in hard copy (paper) form or using the MY AGREE PLUS platform for electronic appraisal, which allows individual appraisals, group appraisals, and group comparisons.

Instructions are provided on the first pages of the instrument. Review and critique can be done individually and compared as a group for team decision-making.

AGREE Enterprise website:

http://www.agreetrust.org/agree-ii

AGREE II online training tools:

http://www.agreetrust.org/resource-centre/agree-ii-training-tools

AGREE publications about the instrument:

http://www.agreetrust.org/resource-centre/key-articles-agree-instrument

AGREE II user manual and instrument:

http://www.agreetrust.org/wp-content/uploads/2013/10/AGREE-II-Users-Manual-and-23-item-Instrument_2009_UPDATE_2013.pdf

MY AGREE PLUS platform for electronic appraisal:

Video: http://www.agreetrust.org/2013/06/important-website-upgrade

Platform:

http://www.agreetrust.org/login/?redirect_to=http%3A%2F%2Fwww.agreetrust.org%2Fmy-agree%2F

(AGREE Collaboration, 2010)

Tool 5.6   Appraise Evidence

INSTRUCTIONS: Determine the kind of evidence being reviewed and associated resources. Link into each and select a resource that best meets the needs of the team.

Organization	Content or Purpose	Website
Multiple Tools		
Critical Appraisal Skills Programme	Critical appraisal skills training, workshops, and tools	http://www.casp-uk.net
Centre for Evidence-Based Medicine, University of Oxford	CEBM tools, examples, and downloads for the critical appraisal of medical evidence	http://www.cebm.net/index.aspx?o=1157
International Centre for Allied Health Evidence	A list of critical appraisal tools, linked to the websites where they were developed	http://www.unisa.edu.au/Research/ Sansom-Institute-for-Health-Research/ Research/Allied-Health-Evidence/ Resources/CAT
Institute of Medicine	Book available online or as paperback. Describes standards for scholarly systematic reviews to help developers and reviewers	http://nationalacademies.org/hmd/ reports/2011/finding-what-works-in-health-care-standards-for-systematic-reviews.aspx _or_ http://nationalacademies.org/hmd/ reports/2015/decreasing-the-risk-of-developing-alzheimers-type-dementia. aspx
Systematic Reviews		
Assessment of Multiple Systematic Reviews, EMGO Institute, The Netherlands	AMSTAR tool for assessing the methodological quality of systematic reviews	https://amstar.ca/Amstar_Checklist.php
British Medical Journal Clinical Evidence	BMJ framework for assessing systematic reviews	http://clinicalevidence.bmj.com/x/set/ static/ebm/toolbox/665052.html
Ottawa Hospital Research Institute	Framework and tools for creating systematic reviews	http://www.prisma-statement.org/
Institute of Medicine	Book available online or as paperback. Describes standards for scholarly systematic reviews to help developers and reviewers	http://nationalacademies.org/hmd/ reports/2011/finding-what-works-in-health-care-standards-for-systematic-reviews.aspx _or_ http://nationalacademies.org/hmd/ reports/2015/decreasing-the-risk-of-developing-alzheimers-type-dementia. aspx

Clinical Practice Guidelines		
The Appraisal of Guidelines for Research and Evaluation Enterprise	A generic tool (AGREE II) for evaluating the quality of reporting and quality of recommendations	http://www.agreetrust.org/agree-ii
Institute of Medicine	Book available online or as paperback. Describes standards for scholarly clinical practice guidelines to help developers and reviewers	http://www.nationalacademies.org/hmd/Reports/2011/Clinical-Practice-Guidelines-We-Can-Trust.aspx
Institute for Quality and Efficiency in Health Care (IQWiG), Cologne, Germany	A systematic review to identify and compare appraisal tools	http://journals.plos.org/plosone/article?id=10.1371/journal.pone.0082915
Tools for Rating Evidence		
U.S. Preventive Services Task Force	USPSTF grades three things: quality of the overall body of evidence, strength of evidence and magnitude of benefit for recommendations, and certainty of outcomes	http://www.uspreventiveservicestaskforce.org/Page/Name/methods-and-processes#recommendation-process
Grading of Recommendations Assessment, Development, and Evaluation	An informal working group whose members have developed a common, sensible, and transparent approach to grading quality of evidence and strength of recommendations	http://www.gradeworkinggroup.org

TOOLS

Tool 5.7 Systematic Review Appraisal

INSTRUCTIONS: Write in enough citation information to locate the article again later. Skip to "critique" section in the middle of page one. Answer each question. Return to the "overall evaluation" section for final consideration of the whole document. Answer the questions in the "overall evaluation" section and determine if the document will be used as part of the body of evidence or discarded.

Citation

Nugent B, Lewis S, O'Sullivan JM, Enteral feeding methods for nutritional management in patients with head and neck cancers being treated with radiotherapy &/or chemotherapy. Cochrane Database of Systematic Reviews 2013, Issue 1. Art. No.: CD007904. DOI: 10.1002/14651858.CD007904.pub3. Accessed 02 April 2021

Overall Evaluation (provide answers after completing the critique)

Internal validity: Does it provide a precise and unbiased answer to the research question?	☐ Totally adequate ☑ Moderately adequate ☐ Not adequate ☐ Can't tell
External validity: Can findings be applied to the population and setting of the EBP initiative?	☑ Totally adequate ☐ Moderately adequate ☐ Not adequate ☐ Can't tell
Are limitations and biases reported and controlled adequately to include this study in the body of evidence for the EBP initiative?	☑ Yes ☐ No
Are inclusion (and no exclusion) criteria met for EBP initiative?	☑ Yes ☐ No

Critique

Background

Is the need for a systematic review clear?	☑ Yes ☐ No
Does the need for a systematic review stem from a clinical problem?	☑ Yes ☐ No
Is the background literature relevant to the problem?	☑ Yes ☐ No

Aim or Objective of the Report

Are elements of PICO (Patient population/problem/pilot area, Intervention, Comparison, and Outcome) discernible?	☑ Yes ☐ No
Is a question about practice clearly written with a focused direction for designing the analysis?	☑ Yes ☐ No
Will the answer to the question provide direction for the clinical problem?	☐ Yes ☑ No

Search Strategies

Are the databases searched appropriate for the aim or objective?	☐ Yes ☑ No
Are the search strategies logical and inclusive?	☑ Yes ☐ No

TOOLS

Search Strategies (Continued)

Is the search process transparent and reproducible?	☒ Yes ☐ No
Is the search yield sufficient for informing clinical practice?	☒ Yes ☐ No
Are inclusion and exclusion criteria clear?	☒ Yes ☐ No
Is the approach to addressing discrepancies clear?	☐ Yes ☒ No

Methods

Do at least two independent reviewers determine inclusion or exclusion of studies?	☒ Yes ☐ No
Are characteristics of the included studies provided?	☒ Yes ☐ No
Is the quality of the studies assessed and used appropriately in forming conclusions?	☒ Yes ☐ No
Are statistical methods for combining results appropriate for the data?	☐ Yes ☒ No
Are qualitative methods used to supplement quantitative methods?	☒ Yes ☐ No

Results/Implications

Are limitations and biases identified?	☒ Yes ☐ No
Are conflicts of interest identified?	☒ Yes ☐ No
Do the results provide direction for the clinical problem?	☐ Yes ☒ No
Are conclusions appropriate based on the design, analysis, and results presented?	☒ Yes ☐ No
Are recommendations for practice supported by evidence?	☐ Yes ☒ No
Are the recommendations for practice relevant to the EBP initiative?	☒ Yes ☐ No

Notes

Complete the "Overall Evaluation" section at the beginning of this tool.

TOOLS

Tool 5.8   Quantitative Research Appraisal

INSTRUCTIONS: Write in enough citation information to locate the article again later. Skip to "critique" section in the middle of page one. Answer each question. Return to the "overall evaluation" section for final consideration of the whole article. Answer the questions in the "overall evaluation" section and determine if the study will be used as part of the body of evidence or discarded.

Citation

Howes N, Atkinson C, Thomas S, Lewis SJ. Immunonutrition for patients undergoing surgery for head and neck cancer. Cochrane Database of Systematic Reviews 2018, Issue 8. Art.No: CD010964. DOI: 10.1002/14651858. CD010959 pub2. Accessed 02 April 202

Overall Evaluation (provide answers after completing the critique)

Internal validity: Does it provide a precise and unbiased answer to the research question?	☐ Totally adequate ☑ Moderately adequate ☐ Not adequate ☐ Can't tell
External validity: Can findings be applied to the population and setting of the EBP initiative?	☐ Totally adequate ☐ Moderately adequate ☑ Not adequate ☐ Can't tell
Are limitations and biases reported and controlled adequately to include this study in the body of evidence for the EBP initiative?	☑ Yes ☐ No
Are inclusion (and no exclusion) criteria met for EBP initiative?	☑ Yes ☐ No

Critique

Research Question

Are the research questions and/or the study aims clearly stated?	☑ Yes ☐ No
Are the research questions relevant to the EBP initiative?	☑ Yes ☐ No
Do the questions provide direction for the study design?	☑ Yes ☐ No

Literature Review

Are the search strategies clear, logical, and inclusive?	☑ Yes ☐ No
Is current literature related to the research question reported?	☐ Yes ☑ No
Is a gap in knowledge, the need for research, clear?	☑ Yes ☐ No

Method/Design

☐ Randomized controlled trial	☐ Quasi-experimental	☐ Mixed methods
☑ Experimental	☐ Descriptive or observational	☐ Other (specify)

Are the setting and population appropriate for the study question?	☑ Yes ☐ No

©University of Iowa Hospitals and Clinics, Revised June 2017

TOOLS

Method/Design (Continued)

Are the setting and sample similar to the EBP initiative setting and population?	☒ Yes ☐ No
Were statistical methods used to determine a sufficient sample size?	☒ Yes ☐ No
Is group randomization and assignment clear and appropriate for the study question?	☒ Yes ☐ No
Is the rigor of the design sufficient for the study question and existing body of research?	☐ Yes ☒ No
Are the instruments valid and reliable?	☒ Yes ☐ No
Do the instruments used match the study constructs and question?	☒ Yes ☐ No

Data Analysis/Results

Are methods used to prevent, recognize, and control bias?	☒ Yes ☐ No
Is the probability of sampling error identified?	☒ Yes ☐ No
Are the numbers of participants enrolled clearly tracked from the starting sample to analyses?	☒ Yes ☐ No
Are the statistical analyses appropriate for the data and study question?	☒ Yes ☐ No
Are the results clear and understandable?	☒ Yes ☐ No
Do the results reported and interpretation of data match?	☒ Yes ☐ No

Discussion/Implications

Does the discussion match the results?	☒ Yes ☐ No
Is the discussion supported by other relevant research?	☐ Yes ☒ No
Are limitations and threats of bias discussed?	☒ Yes ☐ No
Are implications for application in practice clear and appropriate based on the results?	☒ Yes ☐ No
Are the recommendations for practice relevant to the EBP initiative?	☒ Yes ☐ No

Notes

More research needed to draw an evident correlation/ conclusion

Complete the "Overall Evaluation" section at the beginning of this tool.

Tool 5.9   Qualitative Research Appraisal

INSTRUCTIONS: Write in enough citation information to locate the article again later. Skip to "critique" section in the middle of page one. Answer each question. Return to the "overall evaluation" section for final consideration of the whole article. Answer the questions in the "overall evaluation" section and determine if the study will be used as part of the body of evidence or discarded.

Citation
De Ruysscher D, Faivre-Finn C., Nackaerts K, Jordan K, Arends J, Douillard JY, Ricardi U, Peters S. Recommend for supportive care in patients receiving concurrent chemotherapy and radiotherpy for lung cancer. Ann Oncol. 2020 Jan;31 : 41-49. DOI: 10.1016/j.annonc.2019.10.003. PMID: 31912794

Overall Evaluation (provide answers after completing the critique)	
Trustworthiness: Are credibility and confidence in the true value established? Are the results an accurate reflection of the participants' experience?	☑ Totally adequate ☐ Moderately adequate ☐ Not adequate ☐ Can't tell
Applicability: Can findings be applied to the population and setting of the EBP initiative?	☐ Totally adequate ☑ Moderately adequate ☐ Not adequate ☐ Can't tell
Are the methods consistent (dependable) and neutral (confirmable) so as to include this study in the evidence for this EBP initiative?	☑ Yes ☐ No
Are inclusion (and no exclusion) criteria met for the EBP initiative?	☐ Yes ☑ No

Critique	
Topic/Purpose	
Is the phenomenon of interest (topic) clear?	☑ Yes ☐ No
Is the purpose of the study clear?	☑ Yes ☐ No
Do the research questions provide direction for a qualitative design?	☑ Yes ☐ No
Is the topic relevant to the EBP initiative?	☐ Yes ☐ No

Method/Design

☑ Observation   ☐ Triangulation   ☐ Other (specify)
☑ Comparative   ☐ Mixed methods

Is sampling appropriate for the method?	☐ Yes ☑ No
Do participants have an insider's view of the topic?	☑ Yes ☐ No
Do the design and methods fit the study purpose?	☑ Yes ☐ No

Method/Design (Continued)

Are methods well described and replicable?	☐ Yes ☒ No
Is data collection focused on the participants' experience?	☒ Yes ☐ No

Data Analysis/Results

Are the numbers of participants enrolled clearly tracked from the starting sample to analyses?	☐ Yes ☒ No
Are analyses appropriate for the study question and data?	☐ Yes ☒ No
Are data collection and methods dependable (i.e., executed consistently)?	☐ Yes ☒ No
Are analysis methods and results confirmable (i.e., tracked and documented)?	☐ Yes ☒ No
Do methods and results accurately reflect the participants' experience?	☒ Yes ☐ No
Are analyses adequately validated (e.g., triangulation)?	☐ Yes ☒ No
Are the methods and results credible?	☐ Yes ☒ No
Do results add meaning or understanding to the EBP initiative?	☒ Yes ☐ No
Are findings applicable to the patients in the EBP initiative?	☒ Yes ☐ No

Discussion/Implications

Does the report read like a narrative (i.e., telling a story)?	☒ Yes ☐ No
Are the findings reported in context?	☒ Yes ☐ No
Are findings supported by other relevant research?	☒ Yes ☐ No
Are the implications for practice clear?	☒ Yes ☐ No
Are the implications for practice relevant to the EBP initiative?	☒ Yes ☐ No

Notes

Complete the "Overall Evaluation" section at the beginning of this tool.

Tool 5.10   Other Evidence Appraisal

INSTRUCTIONS: Write in enough citation information to locate the document again later. Skip to "critique" section in the middle of page one. Answer each question. Return to the "overall evaluation" section for final consideration of the whole document. Answer the questions in the "overall evaluation" section and determine if the report will be used as part of the body of evidence or discarded.

Citation

Medvec B, Esophageal Cancer: Treatment and Nursing Interventions. Semin oncol Nursing 1988 Nov; 4(4): 246-56. DOI: 10.1016/0749-2081 (88) 90076-9. PMID: 3060921

Overall Evaluation (provide answers after completing the critique)

Internal validity: Does it provide a precise and unbiased answer to the clinical question?	☐ Totally adequate ☐ Moderately adequate ☐ Not adequate ☒ Can't tell
External validity: Can findings be applied to the population and setting of the EBP initiative?	☐ Totally adequate ☐ Moderately adequate ☒ Not adequate ☐ Can't tell
Are limitations and biases reported and controlled adequately to include this in the body of evidence for the EBP initiative?	☐ Yes ☒ No
Are inclusion (and no exclusion) criteria met for the EBP initiative?	☐ Yes ☒ No

Critique

Type of Evidence

Is other evidence limited, indicating a need to expand the pool of evidence, or does this evidence provide a unique perspective?	☐ Yes ☒ No
Is the need for more information clear?	☒ Yes ☐ No
Is this evidence relevant to the problem?	☒ Yes ☐ No
Are scientific principles used?	☐ Yes ☒ No
Are limitations and biases subjectively identified?	☐ Yes ☒ No

Type of Evidence (Continued)

Are conflicts of interest identified?	☐ Yes ☑ No
Is the evidence current (the most recent update has a clear date)?	☐ Yes ☑ No
Do the results provide direction for the clinical problem?	☑ Yes ☐ No
Are conclusions appropriate for the methods and findings presented?	☐ Yes ☑ No
Are recommendations for practice supported by evidence?	☐ Yes ☑ No
Are recommendations for practice relevant to the EBP initiative?	☑ Yes ☐ No

Notes

Complete the "Overall Evaluation" section at the beginning of this tool.

TOOLS

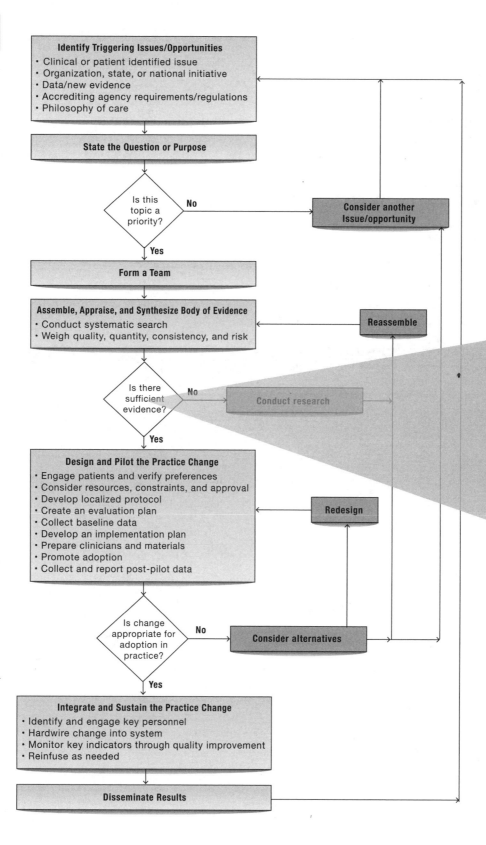

IS THERE SUFFICIENT EVIDENCE?

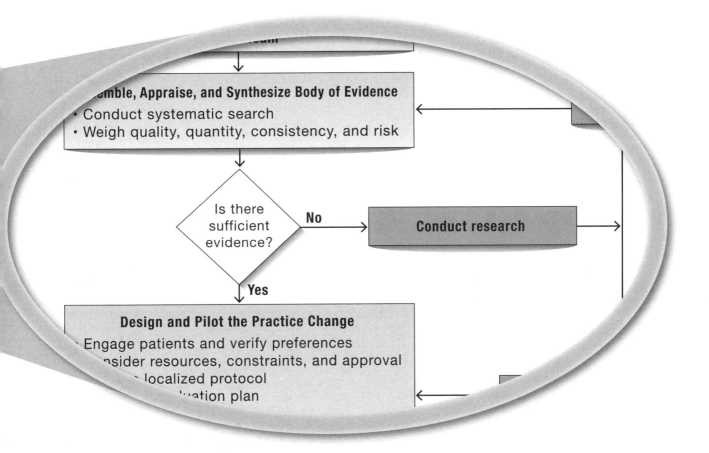

"It is often necessary to make a decision on the basis of information sufficient for action but insufficient to satisfy the intellect."

–Immanuel Kant

At this point, the entire body of evidence—including research, case studies, quality data, expert opinions, and patient input—is synthesized. During this step, the team determines when the evidence is considered sufficient, or not sufficient, for pilot testing.

Tool 6.1   Determine if There Is Sufficient Evidence

INSTRUCTIONS: Review the steps outlined for determining if evidence is sufficient for an EBP change. Identify dates and times for relevant steps, such as meetings to make a list of practice recommendations. Check when steps are completed. Proceed to the next step until each step has been completed.

Date Scheduled	Activity	Done
	Determine the process for analyzing evidence.	☐
	Determine the criteria for making clinical decisions (e.g., strength of evidence, risk, benefit, outcomes).	☐
	Define the key clinical questions and outcomes of interest.	☐
	Review the synthesis table for themes or concepts related to the questions and outcomes of interest.	☐
	Determine the quality and strength of the body of evidence for each question and each outcome.	☐
	Create a list of potential risks for patients associated with the question (e.g., pharmacologic interventions for post-operative pain and slowed return of motility).	☐
	Create a list of potential benefits for patients associated with the question (e.g., pharmacologic interventions for post-operative pain and increased mobility; increased mobility reducing the risk of DVT and pneumonia).	☐
	Draft a list of recommendations for practice, including citations.	☐
	Determine the strength of each recommendation.	☐
	Determine the clinical roles (e.g., nursing, pharmacy) responsible for the recommended practice to ensure that each one is represented in decision-making.	☐
	Convene a team meeting; include additional stakeholders.	☐
	Discuss each potential practice recommendation, the body of evidence supporting the recommendation, and potential risks and benefits.	☐
	Create a project executive summary to concisely update the team and stakeholders; update as project work progresses.	☐

TOOLS

Tool 6.2 Determining Quality Improvement, EBP, or Research

INSTRUCTIONS: Answer each question in the column on the left by checking which box most closely reflects the intent of the work to be accomplished. Review responses as a team. Recognize that all three methods are systematic evaluative methods that include living individuals as part of the evaluation. Discuss and select as a team the method most closely matching the intent. Proceed with relevant notifications and approvals.

	Quality Improvement	Evidence-Based Practice	Research
Which definition fits?	☐ QI is an organizational strategy that formally involves the analysis of process and outcomes data and the application of systematic efforts to improve performance (AHRQ, 2011a). ☐ The degree to which healthcare services for individuals and populations increases the likelihood of desired health outcomes and are consistent with current professional knowledge (IOM, 2004, para. 3).	☐ Evidence-based practice is the process of shared decision-making between practitioner, patient, and others significant to them based on research evidence, the patient's experiences and preferences, clinical expertise or know-how, and other available robust sources of information (STTI, 2008). ☐ Healthcare delivery based on the integration of the best research evidence available combined with clinical expertise, in accordance with the preferences of the patient and family (Sackett et al., 1996; Sackett, Straus, Richardson, Rosenberg, & Haynes, 2000).	☐ Systematic investigation, including research development, testing, and evaluation, designed to develop or contribute to generalizable knowledge; (USDHHS, n.d.-b). ☐ Systematic investigation designed to contribute to generalizable knowledge (USDHHS, n.d.-b).
	Intent		
Who benefits?	☐ Current patients/families ☐ Current clinicians ☐ Organization	☐ Future patients/families ☐ Future clinicians ☐ Organization	☐ Clinicians ☐ Scientific community ☐ Subjects (on occasion)
What is the purpose?	☐ Improve quality or safety of processes or patient experience within the local clinical setting. ☐ Evaluate changes in efficiency or flow.	☐ Improve quality and safety within the local clinical setting by applying evidence in healthcare decisions.	☐ Contribute to and/or generate new knowledge that can be generalized.
What is the scope of interest?	☐ Specific unit or patient population within an organization	☐ Specific unit or patient population within an organization	☐ Generalize to populations beyond organization

	Quality Improvement	Evidence-Based Practice	Research
	Methodology		
Which process or outcome measurements are used?	☐ Measures are simple, easy to use, and administer. ☐ Measures are for key indicators only.	☐ Measures for key indicators using tools with face validity and may be without established validity or reliability. ☐ Measures include knowledge, attitude, behavior/practices, outcomes, and balancing measures (Bick & Graham, 2010; Institute for Healthcare Improvement [IHI], 2017).	☐ Measures are complex. ☐ Increased time is required to fill out the measure. ☐ Measures require a detailed administration plan. ☐ Estimates of reliability, validity, specificity, and/or sensitivity are required.
Which design fits?	☐ Examples include: ☐ Six Sigma ☐ Plan Do Study Act (PDSA) ☐ LEAN ☐ Continuous Quality Improvement (CQI)	☐ Iowa Model or another EBP process model	☐ Randomized control ☐ Quantitative ☐ Qualitative
What is the timing?	☐ Rapid cycle (for example, PDSA)	☐ Planned ☐ Variable timeline based on available clinical practice guidelines or other synthesis reports	☐ Planned and longer
Are there extraneous variables?	☐ Acknowledged but not measured	☐ Acknowledged but not measured	☐ Controlled and/or measured ☐ Tight protocol control
What is the sample?	☐ Convenience sample	☐ Convenience sample	☐ Varied sampling based on study question; may include an established process to improve generalizability of results

continues

Tool 6.2 Determining Quality Improvement, EBP, or Research (Continued)

	Quality Improvement	Evidence-Based Practice	Research
What is the sample size?	☐ Small, but large enough to observe changes ☐ Feasible for data collection	☐ Small, but large enough to observe changes ☐ Feasible for data collection	☐ Size based on estimates of adequate power or saturation
Which data collection is used?	☐ Minimal time, resources, cost	☐ Minimal time, resources, cost	☐ Complex, tightly controlled plan for resources constructed
Which data analysis is used?	☐ Descriptive statistics, run chart, or statistical process control charts for trended data	☐ Descriptive statistics, run chart, or statistical process control charts for trended data; may use inferential statistics	☐ Complex with inferential statistics to promote generalizability of results

Are there relevant regulating bodies?	☐ Organization
	
	 ☐ Influenced by:
	    ☐ The Joint Commission
	    ☐ Centers for Medicare & Medicaid Services
		☐ Organization	☐ Organization, Office of Human Research Protections, FDA, state and local laws

Are there additional burdens or risks?	☐ Patient and/or population is expected to benefit directly from improved flow or process. ☐ Risk of participation is the same as receiving usual clinical care. ☐ If risk or burden is higher than with usual care, consider research and IRB.	☐ Patient and/or population is expected to benefit directly from observations. ☐ Risk of participation is the same as receiving usual clinical care. ☐ If risk or burden is higher than with usual care, consider research and IRB.	☐ Participant is aware of risks. ☐ Informed consent is required. ☐ IRB is required. ☐ Subject may or may not benefit from participation in study.
Is IRB approval needed?	☐ Generally not required unless per organizational policy; recommend checking policy and/or with an organizational leader.	☐ Generally not required when evaluation is limited to QI unless per organizational policy. Recommend a human subject's research determination if there are questions or organization policy/requirements.	☐ Required

	Quality Improvement	Evidence-Based Practice	Research
Is dissemination possible?	☐ Expected to disseminate within the organization; may be expected for public accountability and transparency based on CMS regulations; may be published. ☐ "The intent to publish is an insufficient criterion for determining whether a quality improvement activity involves research. Planning to publish an account of a quality improvement project does not necessarily mean that the project fits the definition of research; people seek to publish descriptions of nonresearch activities for a variety of reasons, if they believe others may be interested in learning about those activities." (USDHHS, n.d.-b, para. 6)	☐ Expected to disseminate within the organization; publication is increasingly becoming an expectation. ☐ Does not indicate generalizability of findings or research (see disseminating quality improvement data). ☐ Adopt SQUIRE 2.0 criteria (Standards for Quality Improvement Reporting Excellence [SQUIRE], 2015)	☐ Expected

CITATIONS

AHRQ, 2011a; Bick & Graham, 2010; IHI, 2017; IOM, 2004; OHRP, 2009; Sackett et al., 1996; Sackett et al., 2000; Sigma Theta Tau International 2005–2007 Research and Scholarship Advisory Committee, 2008; SQUIRE, 2015; USDHHS, n.d.-b.

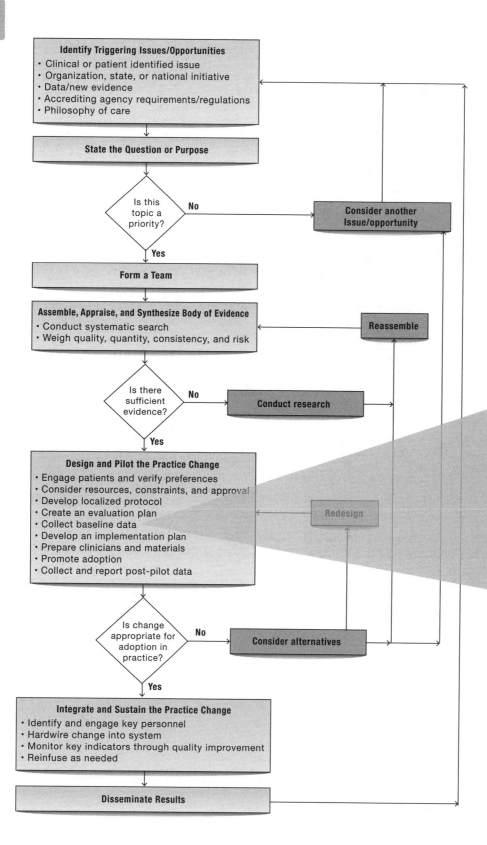

Identify Triggering Issues/Opportunities
• Clinical or patient identified issue
• Organization, state, or national initiative
• Data/new evidence
• Accrediting agency requirements/regulations
• Philosophy of care

State the Question or Purpose

Is this topic a priority?

No → **Consider another Issue/opportunity**

Yes

Form a Team

Assemble, Appraise, and Synthesize Body of Evidence
• Conduct systematic search
• Weigh quality, quantity, consistency, and risk

Reassemble

Is there sufficient evidence?

No → **Conduct research**

Yes

Design and Pilot the Practice Change
• Engage patients and verify preferences
• Consider resources, constraints, and approval
• Develop localized protocol
• Create an evaluation plan
• Collect baseline data
• Develop an implementation plan
• Prepare clinicians and materials
• Promote adoption
• Collect and report post-pilot data

Redesign

Is change appropriate for adoption in practice?

No → **Consider alternatives**

Yes

Integrate and Sustain the Practice Change
• Identify and engage key personnel
• Hardwire change into system
• Monitor key indicators through quality improvement
• Reinfuse as needed

Disseminate Results

DESIGN AND PILOT THE PRACTICE CHANGE

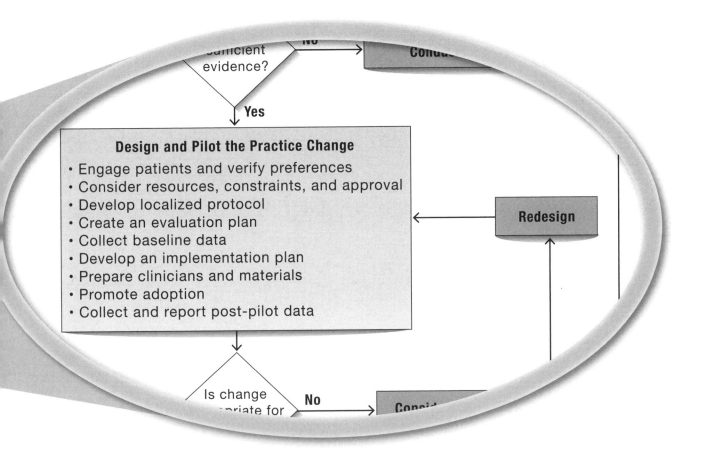

Sufficient evidence?

No → Condu...

Yes ↓

Design and Pilot the Practice Change
- Engage patients and verify preferences
- Consider resources, constraints, and approval
- Develop localized protocol
- Create an evaluation plan
- Collect baseline data
- Develop an implementation plan
- Prepare clinicians and materials
- Promote adoption
- Collect and report post-pilot data

Redesign

Is change ...priate for No → Consi...

"What would life be if we had no courage to attempt anything?"

–Vincent van Gogh

Piloting is an essential step in the EBP process. Outcomes achieved in a controlled research environment may result in different outcomes than those found when EBP is used in a real-world clinical setting. Piloting the EBP change is essential for identifying issues with the intervention, implementation, and potential rollout to multiple clinical areas.

Tool 7.1 Determining a Need for a Policy or Procedure

INSTRUCTIONS: Several considerations would determine the need for a practice policy or procedure. This tool outlines when to consider developing an evidence-based policy or procedure. If any answer is yes, consider developing a practice policy or procedure.

Gap in available policy or procedure on the topic	☐ Yes
	☐ No
Low volume or infrequent patient care issue	☐ Yes
	☐ No
High-risk patient care issue	☐ Yes
	☐ No
Strong commitment to the traditional practice	☐ Yes
	☐ No
Drastic change in practice indicated by current evidence	☐ Yes
	☐ No
Current variation in practice or high probability of variation in practice	☐ Yes
	☐ No
Concern about fidelity of practice change (ability to carry out as intended)	☐ Yes
	☐ No
Variation in practice increases patient risk for poor outcome or increased length of stay	☐ No
	☐ No
Critical steps indicated by current evidence	☐ Yes
	☐ No
Documentation changes needed to support clinicians at the point of care	☐ Yes
	☐ No
New medication or equipment that changes current monitoring or treatments	☐ Yes
	☐ No

TOOLS

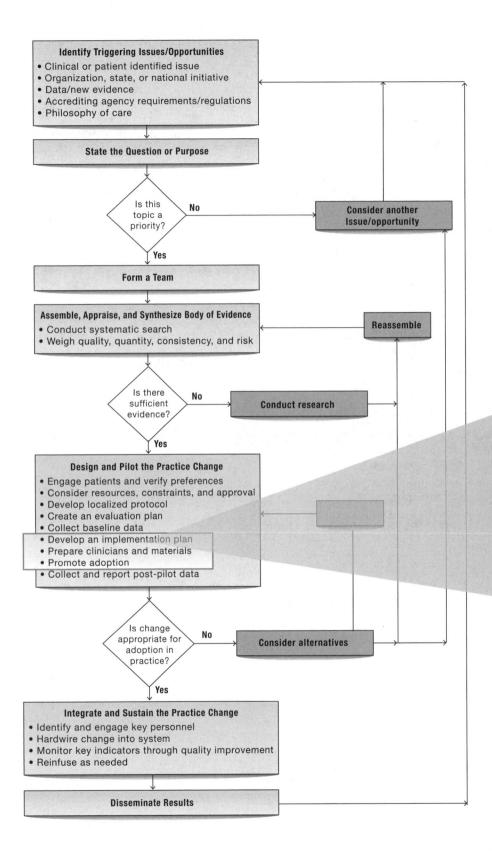

Identify Triggering Issues/Opportunities
- Clinical or patient identified issue
- Organization, state, or national initiative
- Data/new evidence
- Accrediting agency requirements/regulations
- Philosophy of care

State the Question or Purpose

Is this topic a priority?

No → **Consider another Issue/opportunity**

Yes

Form a Team

Assemble, Appraise, and Synthesize Body of Evidence
- Conduct systematic search
- Weigh quality, quantity, consistency, and risk

Reassemble

Is there sufficient evidence?

No → **Conduct research**

Yes

Design and Pilot the Practice Change
- Engage patients and verify preferences
- Consider resources, constraints, and approval
- Develop localized protocol
- Create an evaluation plan
- Collect baseline data
- Develop an implementation plan
- Prepare clinicians and materials
- Promote adoption
- Collect and report post-pilot data

Is change appropriate for adoption in practice?

No → **Consider alternatives**

Yes

Integrate and Sustain the Practice Change
- Identify and engage key personnel
- Hardwire change into system
- Monitor key indicators through quality improvement
- Reinfuse as needed

Disseminate Results

IMPLEMENTATION

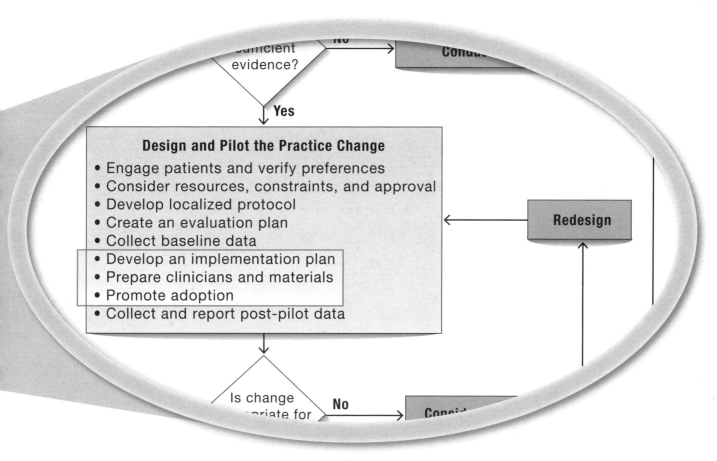

Sufficient
evidence?

No

Condu...

Yes

Design and Pilot the Practice Change
- Engage patients and verify preferences
- Consider resources, constraints, and approval
- Develop localized protocol
- Create an evaluation plan
- Collect baseline data
- Develop an implementation plan
- Prepare clinicians and materials
- Promote adoption
- Collect and report post-pilot data

Redesign

Is change
...priate for

No

Consi...

"A journey of a thousand miles begins with a single step."

–Lao Tzu

Implementation is fluid, complex, and highly interactive, and it changes over the course of the pilot period. Multiple implementation strategies are selected and used cumulatively to create a comprehensive plan based on the four phases of implementation: creating awareness and interest, building knowledge and commitment, promoting action and adoption, and pursuing integration and sustainability (Cullen & Adams, 2012).

TOOLS

Tool 8.1   Selecting Implementation Strategies for EBP

INSTRUCTIONS: Use this worksheet to select strategies and organize an EBP implementation plan. Review considerations outlined in each phase. Add the person responsible, the planned date, and notes for each strategy. Attach this worksheet outlining the implementation plan to the project action plan (see Tool 4.2).

- What are the positive aspects of the EBP?
- Think of this as marketing the EBP.
- Be fun, eye-catching, and memorable.

PHASE 1 CONSIDERATIONS: CREATE AWARENESS AND INTEREST

	Strategies	Resources Needed	Whom to Involve	Date to Initiate
Clinician, Organizational Leaders, and Stakeholders	☐ Highlight advantages or anticipated impact			
	☐ Highlight compatibility			
	☐ Continuing education programs			
	☐ Sound bites			
	☐ Journal club			
	☐ Slogans and logos			
	☐ Staff meetings			
	☐ Unit newsletter			
	☐ Unit inservices			
	☐ Distribute key evidence			
	☐ Posters and postings/fliers			
	☐ Mobile "show on the road"			
	☐ Announcements and broadcasts			
	☐ Knowledge broker(s)			
	☐ Senior executive announcements			
Building Systems	☐ Publicize new equipment			

continues

TOOLS

Tool 8.1   Selecting Implementation Strategies for EBP (Continued)

PHASE 2 CONSIDERATIONS: BUILD KNOWLEDGE AND COMMITMENT

- How do clinicians within a discipline/setting like to learn?
- Build on the natural tendency of clinicians to learn from each other.
- Complete before "go live."

Strategies	Resources Needed	Whom to Involve	Date to Initiate
☐ Education (e.g., live, virtual, or computer-based)			
☐ Pocket guides			
☐ Link practice change and power holder/stakeholder priorities			
☐ Change agents (e.g., change champion, core group, opinion leader, or thought leader)			
☐ Educational outreach or academic detailing			
☐ Integrate practice change with other EBP protocols			
☐ Disseminate credible evidence with clear implications for practice			
☐ Make impact observable			
☐ Gap assessment/gap analysis			
☐ Clinician input			
☐ Local adaptation and simplify			
☐ Focus groups for planning change			
☐ Match practice change with resources and equipment			
☐ Resource manual or materials (i.e., electronic or hard copy)			
☐ Case studies			

Clinician, Organizational Leaders, and Stakeholders

PHASE 2 CONSIDERATIONS: BUILD KNOWLEDGE AND COMMITMENT

Building Systems

- ☐ Teamwork
- ☐ Troubleshoot use/application
- ☐ Benchmark data
- ☐ Inform organizational leaders
- ☐ Report within organizational infrastructure
- ☐ Action plan
- ☐ Report to senior leaders

PHASE 3 CONSIDERATIONS: PROMOTE ACTION AND ADOPTION

- Use highly interactive and personal approaches.
- Demonstrate, encourage return demonstration, and provide reinforcement.
- Keep an eye toward building the EBP into the system and to make it easy to do it right.

Clinician, Organizational Leaders, and Stakeholders

Strategies	Resources Needed	Whom to Involve	Date to Initiate
☐ Educational outreach/academic detailing			
☐ Reminders or practice prompts			
☐ Demonstrate workflow or decision algorithm			
☐ Resource materials and quick reference guides			
☐ Skill competence			
☐ Give evaluation results to colleagues			
☐ Incentives			
☐ Trying the practice change			
☐ Multidisciplinary discussion and troubleshooting			
☐ "Elevator speech"			

continues

TOOLS

©University of Iowa Hospitals and Clinics, Revised June 2017

Tool 8.1   Selecting Implementation Strategies for EBP (Continued)

PHASE 3 CONSIDERATIONS: PROMOTE ACTION AND ADOPTION (Continued)

	Strategies	Resources Needed	Whom to Involve	Date to Initiate
☐	Data collection by clinicians			
☐	Report progress and updates			
☐	Change agents (e.g., change champion, core group, opinion leader, thought leader)			
☐	Role model			
☐	Troubleshooting at the point of care/bedside			
☐	Provide recognition at the point of care			
☐	Audit key indicators			
☐	Actionable and timely data feedback			
☐	Non-punitive discussion of results			
☐	Checklist			
☐	Documentation			
☐	Standing orders			
☐	Patient reminders			
☐	Patient decision aids			
☐	Rounding by unit and organizational leadership			
☐	Report into quality improvement program			
☐	Report to senior leaders			
☐	Action plan			
☐	Link to patient/family needs and organizational priorities			
☐	Unit orientation			
☐	Individual performance evaluation			

Building Systems

PHASE 4 CONSIDERATIONS: PURSUE INTEGRATION AND SUSTAINED USE

- Think about booster shots or periodic reinfusion.
- Build toward the EBP becoming the norm or the standard way to practice.
- Building EBP into the system is critical to help clinicians.

Clinician, Organizational Leaders, and Stakeholders

Strategies	Resources Needed	Whom to Involve	Date to Initiate
☐ Celebrate local unit progress			
☐ Individualize data feedback			
☐ Public recognition			
☐ Personalize the messages to staff (e.g., reduces work, reduces infection exposure) based on actual improvement data			
☐ Share protocol revisions with clinicians that are based on feedback from clinicians, patient, or family			
☐ Peer influence			
☐ Update practice reminders			

Building Systems

Strategies	Whom to Involve	Date to Initiate	Notes
☐ Audit and feedback			
☐ Report to senior leaders			
☐ Report into quality improvement program			
☐ Revise policy, procedure, or protocol			
☐ Competency metric for discontinuing training			
☐ Project responsibility in unit or organizational committee			
☐ Strategic plan			

TOOLS

continues

TOOLS

Tool 8.1 Selecting Implementation Strategies for EBP (Continued)

PHASE 4 CONSIDERATIONS: PURSUE INTEGRATION AND SUSTAINED USE (Continued)

	Strategies	Whom to Involve	Date to Initiate	Notes
Building Systems	☐ Trend results			
	☐ Present in educational programs			
	☐ Annual report			
	☐ Financial incentives			
	☐ Individual performance evaluation			

Tool 8.2   Collecting Pilot Process Issues

INSTRUCTIONS: This worksheet is to help track successes and problems during the pilot of the EBP change. Use this worksheet throughout each of the implementation phases and add comments and observations as the process unfolds. If needed, add more space to each category to maintain a complete and meaningful record. This will provide valuable information when moving into the "integrate and sustain" step of the EBP process.

QUESTIONS TO KEEP IN MIND

What was the evidence-based change?

How different is the change from existing practice?

How were the pilot units/areas chosen? What criteria were used for selection?

What implementation strategies were used and how effective were they?

What resources were needed to implement the pilot? Were there any difficulties in obtaining those resources?

What policies and/or procedures were affected by the change?

Were there any groups that should have been included in planning the rollout?

Was there variability in the success of the pilot among pilot areas? If so, why?

Was the change adapted at any time during the pilot? If so, why?

continues

TOOLS

Tool 8.2   Collecting Pilot Process Issues (Continued)

Were there any special circumstances that affected the rollout of the pilot (i.e., major changes within the institution such as new patient population, new documentation system, unforeseen leadership or workforce changes)?

How were the outcome indicators chosen?

Were there any difficulties in retrieving outcome data?

Were there any unexpected road blocks to implementing the pilot?

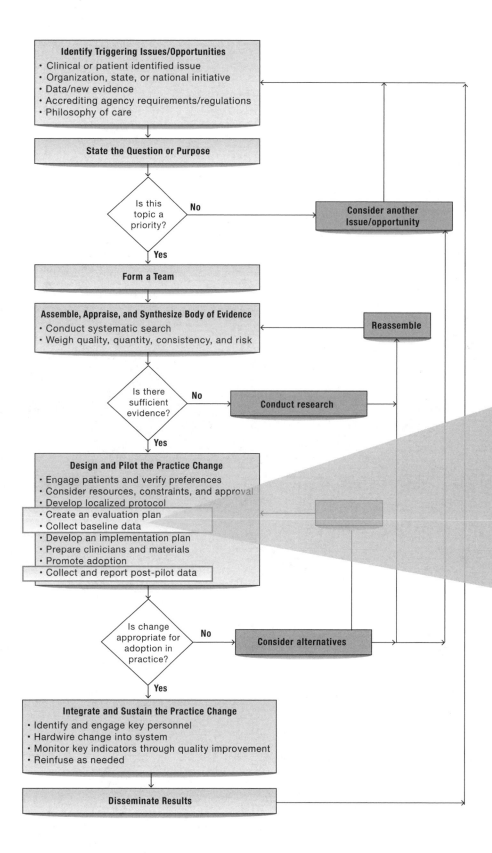

Identify Triggering Issues/Opportunities
- Clinical or patient identified issue
- Organization, state, or national initiative
- Data/new evidence
- Accrediting agency requirements/regulations
- Philosophy of care

State the Question or Purpose

Is this topic a priority?

No → **Consider another Issue/opportunity**

Yes

Form a Team

Assemble, Appraise, and Synthesize Body of Evidence
- Conduct systematic search
- Weigh quality, quantity, consistency, and risk

Reassemble

Is there sufficient evidence?

No → **Conduct research**

Yes

Design and Pilot the Practice Change
- Engage patients and verify preferences
- Consider resources, constraints, and approval
- Develop localized protocol
- Create an evaluation plan
- Collect baseline data
- Develop an implementation plan
- Prepare clinicians and materials
- Promote adoption
- Collect and report post-pilot data

Is change appropriate for adoption in practice?

No → **Consider alternatives**

Yes

Integrate and Sustain the Practice Change
- Identify and engage key personnel
- Hardwire change into system
- Monitor key indicators through quality improvement
- Reinfuse as needed

Disseminate Results

EVALUATION

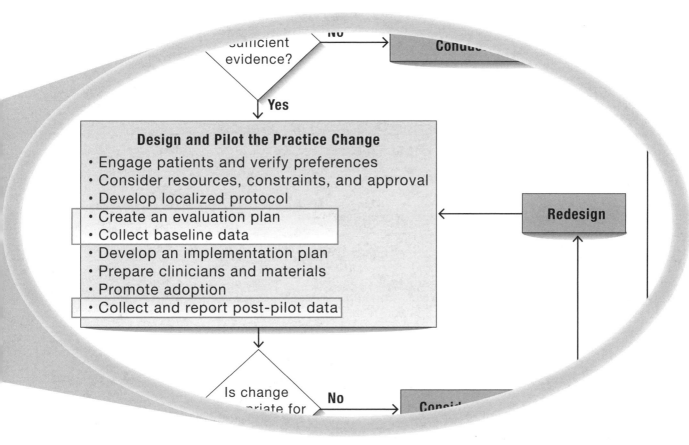

"You may never know what results come of your action, but if you do nothing there will be no result."

–Mahatma Gandhi

Evaluation of the pilot must focus on select key indicators related specifically to the practice change and for input to guide implementation. Both process and outcome indicators are collected before and after implementation of the practice change. A few key indicators will be monitored until the improvement is sustained.

Tool 9.1   Selecting Process and Outcome Indicators

INSTRUCTIONS: Identify key indicators for each of the evaluation components (knowledge, attitude, behavior, outcome, balancing measures). Data collection may be automated if the data are available electronically or may require manual collection.

KNOWLEDGE	
Indicator	**Information to Consider**
Extent of the clinical issue (e.g., incidence, prevalence, rate)	■ Incidence of the problem in the country ■ Rate of an adverse outcome reported in the literature
Gap in local outcome compared to higher performers or in evidence reports	■ Rate of an adverse outcome in the organization, unit, clinic, or setting ■ Rate for higher performers
How to assess the clinical issue	■ Components of an evidence-based assessment ■ Frequency of assessment ■ Tool for assessment and scoring ■ Link between assessment and interventions
Interventions for prevention or treatment	■ Key interventions ■ Location of supplies and how to obtain supplies ■ How to use equipment ■ Precautions for interventions (e.g., patients to exclude, patient risk, how to minimize risk)
Documentation of assessments and interventions	■ Where documentation is available within the documentation system ■ How to differentiate assessment findings for documentation (e.g., pressure injury stages)
PERCEPTION or ATTITUDE	
Indicator	**Example of Wording**
Importance of clinical topic	<Insert clinical topic> is an important clinical issue for patients on my unit.
Relevance of topic to quality and safety	Addressing <insert clinical topic> is a priority for high-quality, safe patient care.
Feeling knowledgeable	I feel knowledgeable in <insert clinical topic>.
Feeling supported	I feel supported in completing <insert clinical topic>.

continues

©University of Iowa Hospitals and Clinics, Revised June 2017

TOOLS

Tool 9.1   Selecting Process and Outcome Indicators (Continued)

PERCEPTION or ATTITUDE

Indicator	Example of Wording
Sufficient time to learn	I have had sufficient time to learn how to complete <insert clinical topic>.
Resources available	<insert clinical topic> resources are readily available for use with patients.
Helpfulness of resource materials	<insert clinical topic> resources are helpful.
Know who can assist	I know who can assist me with <insert clinical topic> care.
Access to an expert	I have ready access to an expert to help troubleshoot the <insert clinical topic> protocol.
Ability to carry out protocol	I am able to carry out the <insert clinical topic> protocol.
Ability to carry out key steps	I am able to carry out key steps in the <insert clinical topic> protocol.
Ease of documentation	Documentation of <insert clinical topic> is easy.

BEHAVIOR or PRACTICE

Indicator	Information to Consider	Data Collection Method
When to evaluate documentation	■ First expected documentation (e.g., within 24 hours of admission) ■ When to evaluate repeated documentation, based on documentation frequency and expected length of stay	■ Chart audit or patient health record report
Documentation by which clinicians	■ Registered nurse ■ Nursing assistant ■ Medical assistant ■ Physician ■ Pharmacist ■ Therapist ■ Nurse practitioner/physician assistant ■ Hospitalist ■ Other	■ Chart audit or patient health record report

Indicator	Information to Consider	Data Collection Method
Key documentation components	▪ Completion of critical variables within <insert clinical topic> ▪ Scoring of variables within <insert clinical topic> ▪ Frequency of each variable within <insert clinical topic> ▪ Completion of patient education ▪ Distribution of patient education materials ▪ Complete key steps within interventions ▪ Frequency of completing key steps within interventions	▪ Chart audit or patient health record report
Current practices	▪ Correct identification of patients for EBP change ▪ Frequency, timing, or completeness of key steps within interventions	▪ Observation ▪ Interview ▪ Self-report
Patient volume or cost	▪ Number of patients who could benefit from the EBP change ▪ Length of stay ▪ Discharge disposition (e.g., improve rate of patients returning home)	▪ Report from billing or EHR

OUTCOMES

Determine where to identify reported outcomes to consider including in the evaluation plan for the EBP change:

▪ Clinical practice guidelines

▪ Research reports

▪ Quality improvement data

▪ Reportable measures

▪ Benchmarks

▪ Organizational data (e.g., length of stay, cost)

BALANCING MEASURES

Determine where to identify outcomes that may conflict with desired outcomes for use in the evaluation plan for the EBP change:

▪ Conflicting research findings

▪ Monitor incident reports of associated risks

▪ Competing practice recommendations

▪ Quality improvement data

▪ Organizational data (e.g., length of stay, cost)

TOOLS

TOOLS

Tool 9.2   Developing Topic-Specific Process and Outcome Indicators

INSTRUCTIONS: Identify key indicators for each of the evaluation components (knowledge, attitude, behavior, outcome, balancing measures). Develop or adapt wording to match topic-specific elements to include in the EBP evaluation.

KNOWLEDGE		
Indicator	**Project-Specific**	**Items to Include**
Extent of the clinical issue (e.g., incidence, prevalence, rate)		☐
Gap in local outcome compared to higher performers or in evidence reports		☐
How to assess the clinical issue		☐
Interventions for prevention or treatment		☐
Where to document assessments and interventions		☐

PERCEPTION or ATTITUDE		
Indicator	**Project-Specific**	**Items to Include**
Importance of clinical topic		☐
Relevance of topic to quality and safety		☐
Feeling knowledgeable		☐
Feeling supported		☐
Sufficient time to learn		☐
Resource materials available		☐
Helpfulness of resource materials		☐
Know who can assist		☐
Access to an expert		☐
Ability to carry out protocol		☐
Ability to carry out key steps		☐
Ease of documentation		☐

BEHAVIOR OR PRACTICE			
Indicator	**Project-Specific**	**Data Collection Method**	**Items to Include**
When to evaluate documentation		☐ Patient chart audit ☐ Patient health record report	☐
Documentation by which clinician(s)	☐ Registered nurse ☐ Nursing assistant ☐ Medical assistant ☐ Physician ☐ Pharmacist ☐ Therapist ☐ Nurse practitioner/ physician assistant ☐ Other	☐ Chart audit ☐ Patient health record report	☐
Key documentation components		☐ Chart audit ☐ Patient health record report	☐
Key components of practice		☐ Observation ☐ Interview ☐ Self-report ☐ Chart audit ☐ Patient health record report	☐
Patient volume or cost		☐ Report from billing ☐ Patient health record report	☐

OUTCOMES				
Sources	**Reported Outcomes**	**Project Data to Obtain**	**Who Can Provide the Data?**	**Items to Include**
Clinical practice guidelines				☐
Research reports				☐
Quality improvement data				☐
Reportable measures				☐
Benchmarks				☐
Organizational data (e.g., length of stay, cost)				☐

continues

TOOLS

TOOLS

Tool 9.2   Developing Topic-Specific Process and Outcome Indicators (Continued)

BALANCING MEASURES				
Sources	Outcomes to Monitor	Project Data to Obtain	Who Can Provide the Data?	Items to Include
Conflicting research findings				☐
Monitor incident reports of associated risks				☐
Competing practice recommendations				☐
Quality improvement data				☐
Organizational data (e.g., length of stay, cost)				☐

NOTE: Select project-specific key indicators for each evaluative component. You must be selective in order to collect relevant data and avoid unnecessary data collection. Select indicators that will help you understand problems and measure changes.

TOOLS

Tool 9.3   Audit Form

INSTRUCTIONS: This tool is designed to audit practice for <topic>. Insert the patient record number and answer each element. Take notes on a separate paper for challenges with identifying data.

Area:

Patient record number:

	Admission/Visit date:	Day1/Visit date:	Day 2/Visit date:
<Insert topic> screening completed by nursing assistant or medical assistant	☐ Yes ☐ No	☐ Yes ☐ No	☐ Yes ☐ No
Clinical changes for <insert symptom> noted	☐ Yes ☐ No	☐ Yes ☐ No	☐ Yes ☐ No
<Insert symptom> documented by nurse, if applicable	☐ Yes ☐ No ☐ Not applicable	☐ Yes ☐ No ☐ Not applicable	☐ Yes ☐ No ☐ Not applicable
<Insert topic> total score	Score: _____	Score: _____	Score: _____
<Insert topic> education documented by nurse	☐ Yes ☐ No	☐ Yes ☐ No	☐ Yes ☐ No
<Insert topic> care interventions documented (or add comment)	☐ <intervention 1> _____ ☐ <intervention 2> _____ ☐ <intervention 3> _____ ☐ <intervention 4> _____ ☐ <intervention 5> _____ ☐ <intervention 6> _____	☐ <intervention 1> _____ ☐ <intervention 2> _____ ☐ <intervention 3> _____ ☐ <intervention 4> _____ ☐ <intervention 5> _____ ☐ <intervention 6> _____	☐ <intervention 1> _____ ☐ <intervention 2> _____ ☐ <intervention 3> _____ ☐ <intervention 4> _____ ☐ <intervention 5> _____ ☐ <intervention 6> _____

Tool 9.4   Clinician Questionnaire

Unit/clinic: _____   **Date:** _____

INSTRUCTIONS: Please take a few minutes to provide valuable feedback related to <topic>. Your responses are anonymous and will be used to improve care for patients with <topic>.

SECTION I: Knowledge assessment

INSTRUCTIONS: Please select the ONE best answer for each question.

1. <insert item>	☐ a. ☐ b. ☐ c. ☐ d.
2. <insert item>	☐ a. ☐ b. ☐ c. ☐ d.
3. <insert item>	☐ a. ☐ b. ☐ c. ☐ d.
4. <insert item>	☐ True ☐ False
5. <insert item>	☐ True ☐ False
6. <insert item>	☐ True ☐ False

SECTION II: Perception or attitude assessment

INSTRUCTIONS: Please indicate the number that best describes your perception or attitude about <topic>.

	Strongly Disagree	Disagree	Agree	Strongly Agree
1. All patients in <clinic/unit> receive <insert topic> care at least <frequency>.	1	2	3	4
2. I am able to identify which patients need to have <insert topic> prevention.	1	2	3	4
3. Using <insert topic or product> enhances the quality of nursing care in the <clinic/unit>.	1	2	3	4
4. I feel knowledgeable about carrying out <insert topic>.	1	2	3	4

SECTION II: Perception or attitude assessment				
	Strongly Disagree	Disagree	Agree	Strongly Agree
5. Completing <insert topic> enables me to meet the health needs of most patients.	1	2	3	4
6. Completing <insert topic> care is important for my patients.	1	2	3	4
7. Informing patients and families about the importance of <insert topic> care is essential for the prevention and reduced severity of <insert outcome>.	1	2	3	4
8. Available patient education materials are helpful in reducing <insert outcome>.	1	2	3	4
9. Documentation of <insert topic> is easy to complete.	1	2	3	4
10. I have easy access to equipment/supplies for providing <insert topic> care.	1	2	3	4
11. I have ready access to experts for assistance providing <insert topic or product> care.	1	2	3	4
12. I feel supported to provide <insert topic> care.	1	2	3	4

TOOLS

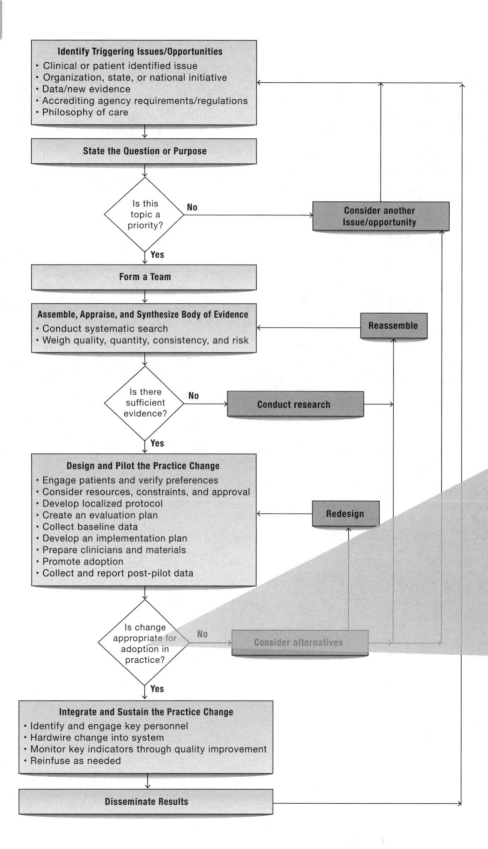

IS CHANGE APPROPRIATE FOR ADOPTION IN PRACTICE?

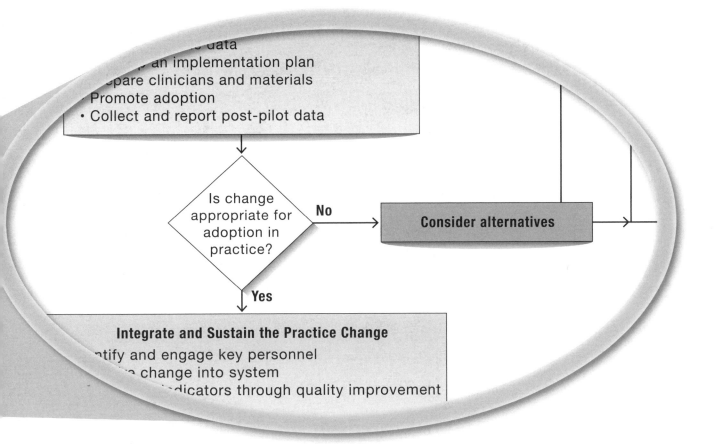

- ... data
- ... an implementation plan
- ...pare clinicians and materials
- Promote adoption
- Collect and report post-pilot data

Is change appropriate for adoption in practice?

No → **Consider alternatives**

Yes

Integrate and Sustain the Practice Change
- ...ntify and engage key personnel
- ... change into system
- ... ...dicators through quality improvement

"Vitality shows in not only the ability to persist, but in the ability to start over."

–F. Scott Fitzgerald

This decision point requires the EBP team to either recommend adoption of the practice change or pursue other courses of action.

Tool 10.1 Decision to Adopt an EBP

INSTRUCTIONS: Insert evaluative data from the pilot. Review results as a team to determine whether evidence-based practice should be adopted as piloted.

KNOWLEDGE

☐ Knowledge pre-data (i.e., total mean percent correct):

☐ Knowledge post-data (i.e., total mean percent correct):

☐ Knowledge improvement (comparing pre-data to post-data):

Sufficient improvement?	☐ Yes ☐ No

If no, describe action needed:

Is mean score > 80%?	☐ Yes ☐ No

Specific items of concern?	☐ Yes ☐ No

If yes, describe problem and solution:

ATTITUDE

Key Indicator/Item	Pre-Data Mean	Post-Data Mean	Change	Threshold Achieved
				☐ Yes ☐ No
				☐ Yes ☐ No
				☐ Yes ☐ No
				☐ Yes ☐ No

*Sample threshold = post-data mean > 3.25; 1–4 scale using Tool 9.4.

BEHAVIOR

Key Indicator/Item	Pre-Data Frequency/Mean	Post-Data Frequency/Mean	Change	Threshold Achieved
				☐ Yes ☐ No
				☐ Yes ☐ No
				☐ Yes ☐ No

*Sample threshold = post-data percent improvement

continues

Tool 10.1   Decision to Adopt an EBP (Continued)

OUTCOMES

Anticipated Outcome #1:	
☐ Outcome pre-data	
☐ Outcome post-data	
Improvement in outcome:	☐ Yes ☐ Not sufficient

If not, describe problem and solution:

Anticipated Outcome #2:	
☐ Outcome pre-data	
☐ Outcome post-data	
Improvement in outcome:	☐ Yes ☐ Not sufficient

If not, describe problem and solution:

Anticipated Outcome #3:	
☐ Outcome pre-data	
☐ Outcome post-data	
Improvement in outcome:	☐ Yes ☐ Not sufficient

If not, describe problem and solution:

Balancing Measure #1:	
☐ Outcome pre-data	
☐ Outcome post-data	
Change in outcome:	☐ Yes ☐ No

If yes, describe problem and solution:

CORRECTIVE ACTION NEEDED

Tool 10.2   EBP Framework for Making Decisions About Adoption of EBP in Practice

INSTRUCTIONS: Read each section and answer questions sequentially. Discuss as a group to determine if the EBP change is appropriate.

1. Do the data suggest that the practice change is better than current practice?

Outcomes and balancing measures data should be used to determine the extent of the benefit (net benefit minus net risk or cost). Decision theory suggests that practice changes resulting in a net benefit should be implemented and that the strength and quality of evidence are irrelevant. However, in real-world clinical settings, the risk of making a wrong decision should be considered.

☐ Yes, change is appropriate ☐ No, consider next question

2. Is the collection of more information worthwhile?

Consider whether the benefit of getting more information outweighs the costs (including time) of collecting it. The value of added information can be determined by these questions:

a. How certain are we of the benefit of the practice change? _____

b. What is the potential impact of a wrong decision? _____

c. Would additional information significantly improve uncertainty? _____

d. What is the cost (including time and lost opportunity for improved outcomes) of collecting more data?
_____

If the value of the information exceeds the costs, it may be worthwhile to consider further pilot testing or research.

☐ No, change is appropriate ☐ Yes, consider next question

3. Should we wait for more evidence?

Consider the risk of implementing now versus waiting, with these questions:

a. How long will it take? _____

b. How likely is it that further evidence will change the practice recommendation? _____

c. What is the cost (e.g., risk) of delaying? _____

d. What would the cost be if the change were implemented and then found to be inferior?
_____

e. Would implementing prevent ongoing testing and future research, or could it be done concurrently?
_____

☐ No, change is appropriate ☐ Yes, consider further pilot testing or research (see Chapter 6)

(Chalkidou, Lord, Fischer, & Littlejohns, 2008)

TOOLS

Tool 10.3　Decision to Implement

INSTRUCTIONS: Determine whether a new clinical tool or process is relevant and worth implementing or adapting for your practice. Use it individually or as a point for team discussion.

1. To what extent do you agree that this intervention:	Strongly Agree	Agree	Disagree	Strongly Disagree
a) Addresses a common or high-priority problem in our practice	1	2	3	4
b) Could be modified to meet the needs of our practice	1	2	3	4
c) Would be simple to implement in our practice	1	2	3	4
d) Is likely to improve processes or patient outcomes in our practice	1	2	3	4
e) Could be pilot tested in our practice prior to fully implementing	1	2	3	4
f) Is relevant to our patient population (from the patient or provider perspective)	1	2	3	4
g) Would work for our patient population	1	2	3	4

2. Consider how you would adopt or adapt this intervention in your practice. What level of resources would you need in the following areas?	Low			High	Don't Know
a) Extent of training for clinicians	1	2	3	4	
b) Changes to workflow, roles, and tasks among team members	1	2	3	4	
c) Technical assistance to modify the patient health record or data systems	1	2	3	4	
d) New and/or additional financial investment/support	1	2	3	4	
e) Support from local practice/clinic leader	1	2	3	4	
3. What is the likelihood that you will adopt or adapt this intervention in your practice in the next year?	1	2	3	4	

4. If you were going to adapt this intervention to your practice, note your ideas about what you would change.

(Research Toolkit, 2013)

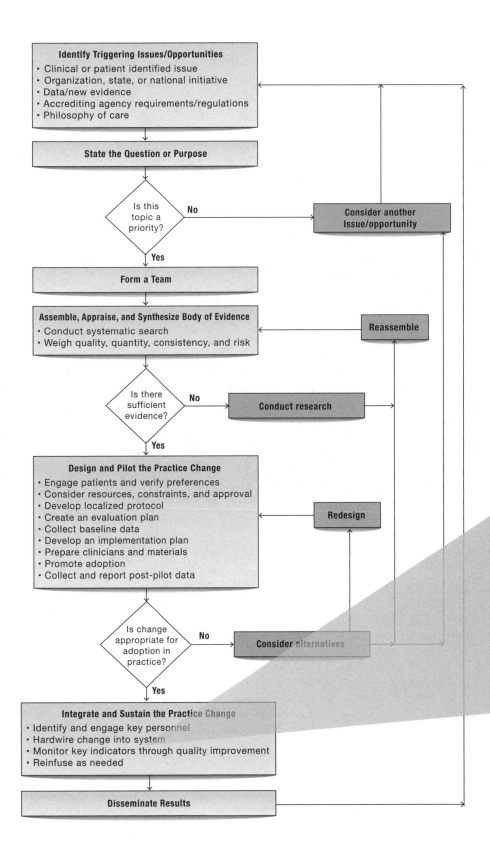

Identify Triggering Issues/Opportunities
- Clinical or patient identified issue
- Organization, state, or national initiative
- Data/new evidence
- Accrediting agency requirements/regulations
- Philosophy of care

State the Question or Purpose

Is this topic a priority?

No → **Consider another Issue/opportunity**

Yes

Form a Team

Assemble, Appraise, and Synthesize Body of Evidence
- Conduct systematic search
- Weigh quality, quantity, consistency, and risk

Reassemble

Is there sufficient evidence?

No → **Conduct research**

Yes

Design and Pilot the Practice Change
- Engage patients and verify preferences
- Consider resources, constraints, and approval
- Develop localized protocol
- Create an evaluation plan
- Collect baseline data
- Develop an implementation plan
- Prepare clinicians and materials
- Promote adoption
- Collect and report post-pilot data

Redesign

Is change appropriate for adoption in practice?

No → **Consider alternatives**

Yes

Integrate and Sustain the Practice Change
- Identify and engage key personnel
- Hardwire change into system
- Monitor key indicators through quality improvement
- Reinfuse as needed

Disseminate Results

INTEGRATE AND SUSTAIN THE PRACTICE CHANGE

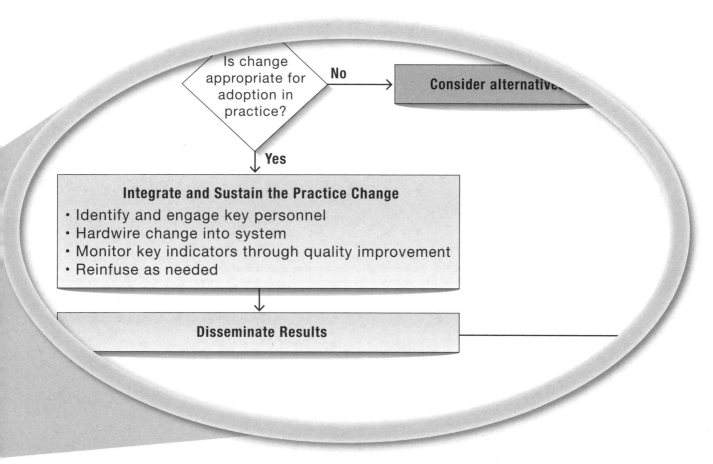

Is change appropriate for adoption in practice?

No →

Consider alternative

Yes

Integrate and Sustain the Practice Change
- Identify and engage key personnel
- Hardwire change into system
- Monitor key indicators through quality improvement
- Reinfuse as needed

Disseminate Results

"If you don't know where you are going, you'll end up somewhere else."

–Yogi Berra

This step promotes integration and sustainability of the practice change over time and prevents regression to previous practice habits. The importance of "hardwiring" the change into the system, tracking evaluative data over time, and planning for periodic reinfusion is emphasized.

THIS PAGE INTENTIONALLY BLANK

Tool 11.1 Action Plan for Sustaining EBP

INSTRUCTIONS: This tool is designed with key steps for integrating and sustaining an EBP change. Review the outlined steps and identify any steps to remove and delete that row. Fill in remaining cells to develop a comprehensive integration plan. Include the key step, specific actions for each step, individuals by name, materials or resources needed, anticipated date for completion, metric to demonstrate completion of the activity, and mark done. Discuss as a team and update regularly.

Project Director Name:	Team:	
Project Purpose: To integrate the _____ EBP practice change into routine workflow as standard practice on _____ (Unit/clinic)		
Key Step or Objective	**Specific Activities to Meet Objective**	**Person Responsible**
Review team membership to focus on integration	Review team membership and determine need to link within shared governance	
	Reconfigure team: Add strategic members	
Internal strategic reporting	Practice/policy committee name: _____	
	Informatics/electronic health record representative _____ (name)	
	Patient education committee _____(name)	
	Staff education committee _____(name)	
	Quality/performance improvement committee _____(name)	
	EBP committee _____(name)	
Identify key data to trend	Identify process indicators with opportunity for improvement	
	Narrow to key process indicators with greatest impact on outcome	
	Identify key outcome indicators	
	Identify balancing measure required to reduced undesired effect, needing ongoing monitoring	
Mobilize QI methods	Generate report within QI/PI system	
	Select appropriate graph to display data trends (e.g., run or statistical process control chart)	

	Materials or Resources Needed	Due Date	Evaluation	Done Date
	Team plan/charter with membership outlined		Updated team membership list	
	Project summary to share		Email and meet/invite	
	Flowchart of committees within shared governance structure		Report project update with proposed policy update	
			Report project update with proposed changes in order sets, documentation, etc.	
			Report project update with proposed patient educational materials with reading level assessment	
			Report project update with proposed plan	
			Report project update with integration plan	
			Report project findings with integration plan	
	Data management resources		Considered knowledge, attitude, and practices/behaviors for clinicians and patients	
			Created list of < 10 indicators for each: knowledge, attitude, and practices/behaviors (see Tools 9.1 and 9.2)	
			Top 2: _____ _____	
			Determined unintended consequence to monitor: _____	
		Quarterly	Example 9.5	
			Histogram for immediate post-pilot (see Tool 11.2)	

continues

Tool 11.1   Action Plan for Sustaining EBP (Continued)

Key Step or Objective	Specific Activities to Meet Objective	Person Responsible
	Monitor data using audit, and report using actionable feedback	
	Identify interprofessional champions for QI cycle	
Select integration strategies	Review Implementation Strategies for EBP	
	Select strategies to continue and to add	
	Determine timing for proactive and regular reinfusion	
	Identify local champion with responsibility to lead through integration	
Set goal	Establish target for integration that indicates change is hardwired	
	Determine when goal is met to remove from future training programs or competency training, if appropriate	
External reporting of lessons learned	Select a venue reaching target audience	
	Choose conference abstract (paper or poster) and/or manuscript	
	Develop and submit an abstract following author guidelines	
Garner continued senior leadership support	Send notification of team success to assist team leaders in recognizing team	
	Report through QI system to senior leaders and board	
	Acknowledge leadership support in success	
Monitor for need to reinvigorate team	Follow trended data for deterioration	
Determine need to cycle back to top of Iowa Model	Identify whether topic work was divided into pieces (e.g., assessment completed first, intervention next)	
	Evidence changes practice recommendation	
	Data indicate deterioration in practice	

Materials or Resources Needed	Timeline	Evaluation	Done Date
		Discipline specific champions: _____	
See Figure 11.2		Team discussion using 15% solutions activity (Lipmanowicz & McCandless, 2014)	
		List strategies with responsibility for follow-up	
	Begin 3 months after pilot evaluation	Quarterly until target reached and sustained for 1 year	
		Clinician champion: _____ _____	
Review pilot evaluation data		Key data meet or exceed goal for 1 year	
		Evaluate quarterly	
		Abstract submission <organization>	
		☐ Paper/oral ☐ Poster	
Expert review before submission		Due <date>	
		Email summary of success	
Brief project/executive summary (see Examples 6.4 and 12.1)		Report project summary	
Example 9.5		Public recognition or send a thank-you note	
		Monitor quarterly	
		Next round will address: <topic>	
		Librarian-assisted search	
		Monitor quarterly	

Tool 11.2   Histograms

INSTRUCTIONS: The procedures for developing, displaying, and interpreting a histogram are outlined as a checklist. Complete each step and mark as each step is done.

Benefits and Limitations

- Easy to understand
- Demonstrates progress toward goal
- Provides an easy-to-identify improvement or need for reinfusion
- Does not indicate if change is normal variation or special cause
- Does not indicate statistical or clinical significance
- Demonstrates static, not dynamic data

Procedure

- ☐ Obtain data software with graphical capability
- ☐ Determine indicators to graph
- ☐ Select frequency of data reporting (e.g., monthly)
  - ○ Determine number of available data points for *x*-axis
- ☐ Select graph: histogram versus run chart or statistical process control chart
  - ○ Consider audience: expertise and preference for data display
  - ○ Use most robust data display option
- ☐ Retrieve or enter data into a spreadsheet or statistical software
- ☐ Plot, arrange, connect data points, and then format data display
  - ○ Maintain full display of *y*-axis end points (e.g., 0–100%)
- ☐ Determine whether a benchmark is available and beneficial to include, add if available
- ☐ Label axis and legends clearly
- ☐ Determine stability or variation in data that indicates whether performance improvement was achieved or intervention is needed
- ☐ Distribute data display with next steps to keep data actionable
- ☐ Consider strategic internal dissemination to executives

Interpreting Histograms

- ☐ Locate the operational definition of the indicator being displayed
- ☐ Consider which measure of central tendency is being displayed (e.g. mean, median)
- ☐ Look for variation
  - ○ Identify the baseline data point
  - ○ Identify the most recent data point

☐ Determine the change from baseline

☐ Determine if improvement is demonstrated in the data (i.e., change in the desired direction)

☐ Determine if goal was achieved and maintained (e.g., more than one post-pilot data point)

☐ Ask questions to expand the understanding of the data

☐ Describe what the data mean, as a story

Example

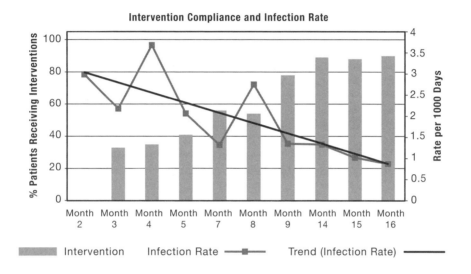

fictitious data

Books and software are listed that provide direction for creating and using histograms.

- Carey, R. G., & Lloyd, R. C. (2001). *Measuring quality improvement in healthcare: A guide to statistical process control applications.* Milwaukee, WI: ASQ Quality Press.

- KhanAcademy. (2016). Creating a histogram [Video file]. Retrieved from https://www.khanacademy.org/math/cc-sixth-grade-math/cc-6th-data-statistics/histograms/v/histograms-intro

- Microsoft. (n.d.). Create a histogram. Retrieved from https://support.office.com/en-us/article/Create-a-histogram-B6814E9E-5860-4113-BA51-E3A1B9EE1BBE

- MySecretMathTutor. (2011, September 1). Statistics–how to make a histogram [Video file]. Retrieved from https://www.youtube.com/watch?v=KCH_ZDygrm4

- Smith, J. M. (2014). *Meaningful graphs: Converting data into informative Excel® charts.* United States of America: Author.

- Statistics How To. (2013). Make a histogram in easy steps. Retrieved from http://www.statisticshowto.com/make-histogram

Tool 11.3   Run Charts

INSTRUCTIONS: The procedures for developing, displaying, and interpreting a run chart are outlined as a checklist. Complete each step and mark as each step is done. Use the examples as a visual tool.

Benefits and Limitations

- Demonstrates progress toward goal and sustained use of practice improvement

- Easy to identify random vs. non-random change/variation

- Provides an easy-to-identify need for reinfusion

- Improves strength of interpretation by using robust analysis that may demonstrate a clinically significant or statistically significant impact

- Control charts without limits

- Require no statistical calculations

- Easy to understand

- Will not detect all special cause variation

- Require a minimum of 10 data points (although some rules have been extended for use when at least 5 data points are available)

Procedure

- [ ] Obtain data software with graphical capability

- [ ] Determine indicators to graph

- [ ] Select frequency of data reporting (e.g., monthly)
  - ○ Consider audience: expertise and preference for data display
  - ○ Use most robust data display option

- [ ] Select graph: run chart versus histogram, or statistical process control chart

- [ ] Determine number of available data points for *x*-axis

- [ ] Retrieve or enter data into a spreadsheet or statistical software

- [ ] Plot, arrange, connect data points, and then format data display
  - ○ Maintain full display of *y*-axis end points (e.g., 0–100%)

- [ ] Include a median—indicated by a line through the data points

- [ ] Determine whether a benchmark is available and beneficial to include, add if available

- [ ] Label axis and legends clearly

- [ ] Determine stability or variation in data that indicates whether performance improvement was achieved or intervention is needed

TOOLS

☐ Distribute data display with next steps to keep data actionable

☐ Consider strategic internal dissemination to executives

☐ Determine when to freeze the median/mean or limits to demonstrate improvement and/or establish a new goal

Interpreting Run Charts

Use these rules to determine if there is special cause (statistically significant and non-random) as compared to common cause variation (what is usually expected in healthcare data). Data that break these rules indicate special cause variation that requires further investigation.

Rule 1: Identify a shift: six or more consecutive data points above or below the median (ignore the values that fall on the median and continue the count)

☐ If the graph includes fewer than 20 data points (not on the median) then 7 or more equals a shift

☐ If 20 or more data points (not on the median) then 8 or more equals a shift

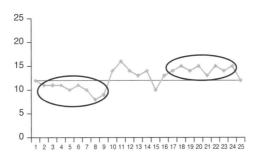

Rule 2: Identify a trend: number of consecutive ascending or descending points; dependent on number of data points. Ignore one of two consecutive data points that are identical.

☐ If there are 5–8 total data points then 5 or more consecutive ascending or descending indicate special cause

☐ If there are 9–20 total data points then 6 or more indicate special cause

☐ If there are 21–100 total data points then 7 or more indicate special cause

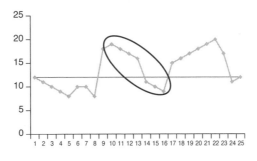

continues

TOOLS

Tool 11.3   Run Charts (Continued)

Interpreting Run Charts (Continued)

__Rule 3__: __Identify a run:__ consecutive data points on the same side of the median. Count number of times the data line crosses the median line AND add one.

☐ Use an established probability to determine whether there are more or fewer than the expected number. (http://www.qihub.scot.nhs.uk/media/529936/run%20chart%20rules.pdf or http://sixsigmastudyguide.com/run-chart)

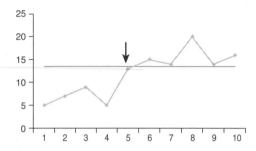

__Rule 4__: __Identify an astronomical point:__ data points that are different from all or a majority of other values as well as being different from the highest and lowest values usually seen

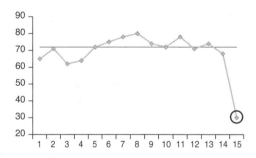

Example

Avdić, A., Tucker, S., Evans, R., Smith, A., & Zimmerman, M. B. (2016). Comparing the ratio of mean red blood cell transfusion episode rate of 1 unit versus 2 units in hematopoietic stem cell transplant patients. *Transfusion, 56*(9), 2346–2351. doi:10.1111/trf.13708

Resources

Books and software are listed that provide direction for creating and using run charts.

- Berardinelli, C., & Yerian, L. (n.d.). Run charts: A simple and powerful tool for process improvement [Web log post]. Retrieved from https://www.isixsigma.com/tools-templates/control-charts/run-charts-a-simple-and-powerful-tool-for-process-improvement

- Blossom, P. (2013, April 1). Create a run chart [Video file]. Retrieved from https://www.youtube.com/watch?v=0FNzoB19G4A

- Carey, R. G., & Lloyd, R. C. (2001). *Measuring quality improvement in healthcare: A guide to statistical process control applications.* Milwaukee, WI: ASQ Quality Press.

- Institute for Healthcare Improvement. (n.d.-a). Run chart tool. Retrieved from http://www.ihi.org/resources/pages/tools/runchart.aspx

- Institute for Healthcare Improvement. (n.d.-b). Whiteboard: Run chart [Video file]. Retrieved from http://www.ihi.org/education/IHIOpenSchool/resources/Pages/AudioandVideo/Whiteboard7.aspx

- National Health Service. (n.d.-c). Run chart rules for interpretation. Retrieved from http://www.qihub.scot.nhs.uk/media/529936/run%20chart%20rules.pdf

- Perla, R. J., Provost, L. P., & Murray, S. K. (2011). The run chart: A simple analytical tool for learning from variation in healthcare processes. *BMJ Quality & Safety, 20*(1), 46–51. doi:10.1136/bmjqs.2009.037895.

- Six Sigma study guide. ((2014, January 20). Run chart: Creation, analysis, & rules. Retrieved from http://sixsigmastudyguide.com/run-chart

- Smith, J. M. (2014). *Meaningful graphs: Converting data into informative Excel® charts.* United States of America: Author.

Tool 11.4   Statistical Process Control Charts

INSTRUCTIONS: The procedures for developing, displaying, and interpreting a statistical process control chart are outlined as a checklist. Complete each step and mark as each step is done. Use the examples as a visual tool.

Benefits and Limitations

- Demonstrates progress toward goal and sustained use of practice improvement
- Easy to identify random vs. non-random change/variation
- Provides an easy-to-identify need for reinfusion
- Improves strength of interpretation by using robust analysis that may demonstrate a clinically significant or statistically significant impact
- Will not detect all special cause variation
- Requires a minimum of 15 data points

Procedure

- ☐ Obtain data software with graphical capability
- ☐ Determine indicators to graph
- ☐ Select frequency of data reporting (e.g., monthly)
  - ○ Consider audience: expertise and preference for data display
  - ○ Use most robust data display option
- ☐ Select graph: statistical process control chart versus histogram or run chart
- ☐ Determine number of available data points for *x*-axis
- ☐ Determine whether displaying continuous or discrete data and select the type of chart to use
- ☐ Retrieve or enter data into a spreadsheet or statistical software
- ☐ Plot, arrange, connect data points, and then format data display
  - ○ Maintain full display of *y*-axis end points (e.g., 0–100%)
- ☐ Include a mean—indicated by a line through the data points
- ☐ Determine whether a benchmark is available and beneficial to include, add if available
- ☐ Label axis and legends clearly
- ☐ Determine stability or variation in data that indicates whether performance improvement was achieved or intervention is needed
  - ○ Mark the time points on the graph when interventions occurred.

TOOLS

○ Look for common cause and special cause variation. Common cause variation is expected and is the usual variation seen in real life (e.g., time needed to go from home to work varies). Special cause variation is a statistically significant change in trended data (e.g., construction or an accident significantly interfering with your travel time between home and work). Identify special cause variation by using the seven rules outlined in the section that follows.

○ Note that an improvement from an EBP change in practice procedures may shift the mean or create a positive special cause variation that is in the desired direction (e.g., significantly fewer hospital-acquired events).

☐ Identify key components of the graph:

○ Find the mean, indicated by a line through the center of the data points on the graph.

○ Identify Zone C: First locate the mean. Then locate the first line on either side of the mean. Zone C is one sigma or approximately one standard deviation away from the mean. Sigma is used to indicate data spread. If the data are normally distributed (i.e., bell-shaped curve), Zone C will contain about 68% of the data points.

○ Next identify Zone B: This is approximately two standard deviations on either side of the mean. If the data are normally distributed, Zone B will contain about 95% of the data points.

○ Lastly identify Zone A: This is approximately three standard deviations on either side of the mean. Zone A will contain 99% of the data, if data are normally distributed.

○ Upper control limit (UCL) is three sigmas (or standard deviations) above the mean. The UCL may be displayed with a static or roving line on the upper edge of Zone A.

○ Lower control limit (LCL) is three sigmas below the mean. The LCL will be displayed with a static or roving line, matching the UCL, and is located on the lower edge of Zone A. In healthcare the LCL may be zero and not included on the graph.

○ In some cases, only the three sigmas or UCL and LCL will be displayed because they are fairly easily applied in practice.

☐ Distribute data display with next steps to keep data actionable

☐ Consider strategic internal dissemination to executives

☐ Determine when to freeze the mean or limits to demonstrate improvement and/or establish a new goal

continues

Tool 11.4   Statistical Process Control Charts (Continued)

Interpreting Statistical Process Control Charts

INSTRUCTIONS: Use these rules to determine if there is special cause (statistically significant and non-random) as compared to common cause variation (what is usually expected in healthcare data). Data that break these rules indicate special cause variation that requires further investigation.

■ **Rule 1: Beyond Limits:** Any point beyond Zone A

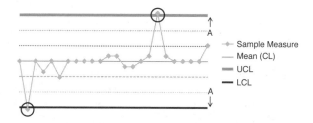

■ **Rule 2: Zone A:** Two of three consecutive points in Zone A or beyond

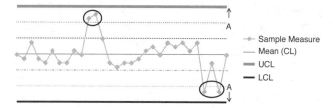

■ **Rule 3: Zone B:** Four of five data points in Zone B or beyond on the same side of the center line

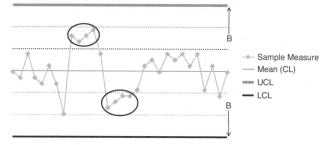

■ **Rule 4: Zone C:** Eight consecutive data points on either side of the center line in Zone C or beyond

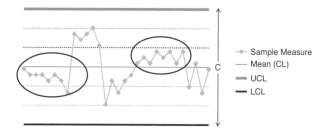

■ **Rule 5: Trend:** Six or more data points steadily increasing or decreasing

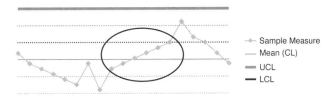

■ **Rule 6: Over-Control:** Fourteen consecutive data points alternating up and down (sawtooth pattern)

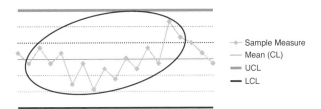

■ **Rule 7: Stratification:** Fifteen consecutive data points within Zone C

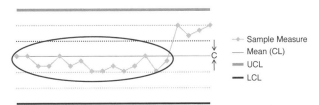

Example

Fisher, D., Cochran, K., Provost, L., Patterson, J., Bristol, T., Metzguer, K., ... McCaffrey, M. (2013). Reducing central line-associated bloodstream infections in North Carolina NICUs. *Pediatrics, 132*(6), 1–8. doi:10.1542/peds.2013-2000

continues

TOOLS

Tool 11.4   Statistical Process Control Charts (Continued)

Resources

Articles, books, and online resources are listed that provide direction for creating and using statistical process control charts.

- Benneyan, J. C., Lloyd, R. C., & Plsek, P. E. (2003). Statistical process control as a tool for research and healthcare improvement. *Quality & Safety in Health Care, 12*(6), 458–464.

- Carey, R. G., & Lloyd, R. C. (2001). *Measuring quality improvement in healthcare: A guide to statistical process control applications.* Milwaukee, WI: ASQ Quality Press.

- Institute for Health Improvement [IHI Open School]. (2014a, May 5). Whiteboard: Control charts [Video file]. Retrieved from https://www.youtube.com/watch?v=9kmblj5zRtA

- Institute for Health Improvement [IHI Open School]. (2014b, May 5). Whiteboard: Static vs. dynamic data [Video file]. Retrieved from https://www.youtube.com/watch?v=UJqvC_uo63M

- Mohammed, M. A., Worthington, P., & Woodall, W. H. (2008). Plotting basic control charts: Tutorial notes for healthcare practitioners. *Quality & Safety in Health Care, 17*(2), 137–145. doi:10.1136/qshc.2004.012047

- National Health Service. (n.d.-a). Quality and service improvement tools: Statistical process control (SPC). Retrieved from http://webarchive.nationalarchives.gov.uk/20121108103848/http://www.institute.nhs.uk/quality_and_service_improvement_tools/quality_and_service_improvement_tools/statistical_process_control.html

- National Health Service. (n.d.-b). Quality and service improvement tools: Variation—an overview. Retrieved from http://webarchive.nationalarchives.gov.uk/20121108105624/http://www.institute.nhs.uk/quality_and_service_improvement_tools/quality_and_service_improvement_tools/variation_-_an_overview.html

- National Health Service. (2010). Explanation of statistical process control charts: Changes to the presentation of information in the *Staphylococcus aureus* bacteremia quarterly reports. Retrieved from http://www.wales.nhs.uk/sites3/page.cfm?orgid=379&pid=13438

- Schmaltz, S. (2011). A selection of statistical process control tools used in monitoring health care performance. Rockville, MD: Agency for Healthcare Research and Quality. Retrieved from http://qualitymeasures.ahrq.gov/expert/expert-commentary.aspx?id=16454

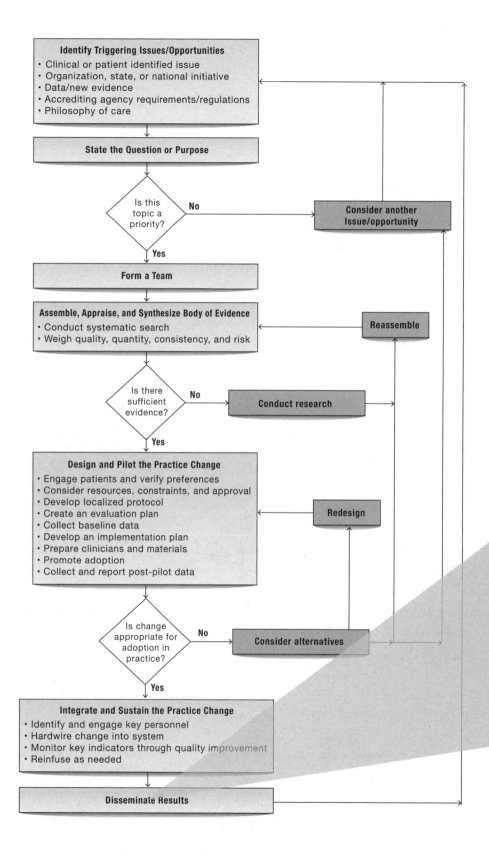

DISSEMINATE RESULTS

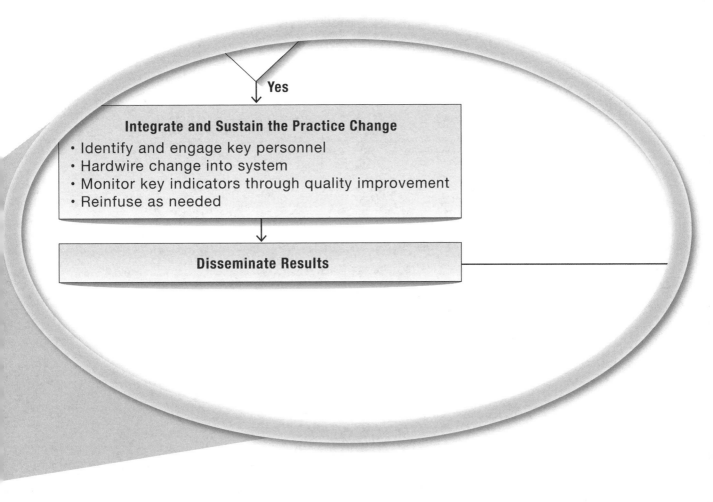

Yes

Integrate and Sustain the Practice Change
- Identify and engage key personnel
- Hardwire change into system
- Monitor key indicators through quality improvement
- Reinfuse as needed

Disseminate Results

"If opportunity doesn't knock, build a door."

–Milton Berle

Dissemination of project results is a key step in the EBP process to promote the adoption of EBPs within the larger healthcare community (Sigma Theta Tau International 2005–2007 Research and Scholarship Advisory Committee, 2008). Sharing project reports within and outside the organization through presentation and publication supports the growth of an EBP culture in the organization, expands nursing knowledge, and encourages EBP updates in other settings.

Tool 12.1 Creating an EBP Poster

INSTRUCTIONS: Creating a poster is an easy way to share information about your EBP project. Refer to the checklist for elements to include in a poster presentation. The poster should be created for readability and focused on key messages.

☐ Use a large font size (> 28).

☐ Be inclusive when listing interprofessional team members of the EBP project.

☐ Consider the following components:

- Project title
- Interprofessional team members' names and credentials
- Purpose statement
- Rationale or background (optional)
- Project framework or EBP process
- Synthesis of evidence
- Practice change
- Implementation strategies
- Evaluation or results
- Next steps
- Conclusions and implications for practice

☐ Place content in columns; readers will read down each column and from left to right.

☐ Credit the funding agency, if applicable.

☐ Use color and images to enhance the story without overdoing it.

☐ Report data in graphs with minimal text for easy interpretation.

☐ Label graphs and legends clearly (e.g., label x and y axes, note sample size).

☐ Provide a link to the program or conference theme, if applicable.

CITATIONS

American Nurses Association, 2009; Forsyth, Wright, Scherb, & Gaspar, 2010; Hanrahan, Marlow, Aldrich, & Hiatt, 2012; Siedlecki, 2017; Williams & Cullen, 2016.

Tool 12.2   Institutional Review Board Considerations

INSTRUCTIONS: It may be unclear whether EBP work should have Institutional Review Board (IRB) review and approval. This tool provides a checklist of resources and forms to locate within your organization. When questions emerge, seek assistance from an organizational leader and/or EBP expert.

IRB Review Resources

☐ Chair or members of the Nursing Research and EBP Committee

☐ Clinical IRB chair (can help differentiate EBP from conduct of research)

☐ Organizational policies

☐ Office for Human Research Protections: http://www.hhs.gov/ohrp

IRB Review and Form Completion

☐ Always follow institutional policies regarding IRB review for QI.

☐ Regular discussions about the approval process between the group responsible for EBP work and the clinical IRB chair may be helpful.

☐ Complete a Human Subjects Research Determination request form for review by the institutional IRB clinical chair.

☐ When completing the Human Subjects Research Determination request form, use concise QI language instead of research terms:

- QI/EBP project director (not *principal investigator*)

- Describe practice change (not *intervention*)

- Evaluation plan (not *methodological design*)

☐ If project results are sensitive, consider reporting in a manner that provides more general outcomes (e.g., a decrease in fall rate by X% instead of a fall rate reduction from X/1000 patient days to Y/1000 patient days).

Tool 12.3   EBP Abstract Template

INSTRUCTIONS: Read carefully and follow directions for the conference or program. Include a brief summary of the EBP project-specific information in each section identified. Include all sections in the outline, per call for abstracts directions for specific format and word limits.

Project Title:

Author(s):

Purpose and Rationale: Clearly state the project purpose (include PICO [P = patient population/problem/pilot area, I = intervention, C = comparison, O = outcome] components within the purpose statement) and the rationale for doing the project.

Synthesis of Evidence: Provide a synthesis of the available evidence (i.e., not an annotated bibliography).

_____

Practice Change: Explain the practice change as a procedure that can be replicated.

_____

Implementation Strategies: Describe implementation strategies used to introduce and integrate the change in practice.

_____

Evaluation: Describe the evaluation used or planned for the project. Report findings related to both process and outcome indicators.

_____

Conclusions and Implications for Practice: Summarize the project findings and how they might be used in practice.

_____

References:

_____

Total Words/Figures Allowed:

TOOLS

Tool 12.4 Preparing an EBP Presentation

INSTRUCTIONS: Review the checklist and conference directions carefully. Follow each step, checking when complete. Include all elements in the presentation.

- [ ] Carefully read the specifications for the presentation, especially if there is a required or recommended program to use.

- [ ] Know your presentation time limit. A general rule of thumb is to plan to cover one slide in two minutes.

- [ ] Determine what equipment will be provided and notify the sponsoring organization of any special equipment needs, such as access to the Internet or sound.

- [ ] Select a template or design style and use a consistent design style, font style, and font sizes throughout.

- [ ] Create a title slide with byline, institutional logos, and sponsorship (such as grants or other paid endorsements), as appropriate.

- [ ] Report any conflict of interest or intellectual bias.

- [ ] Identify objectives or an outline for the presentation.

- [ ] Identify the key pieces of information you want the audience to learn. Do not bombard the audience with every detail about the project.

- [ ] Use slide titles to inform participants of the pertinence of the content on that slide.

- [ ] Use well-labeled graphs when possible; graphs are easier to read than tables.

- [ ] When adding tables, figures, or images, keep objects proportional (avoid distortion).

- [ ] Include authors' last name and the year of publication for direct citations or specific research studies:

    - ○ Cite directly on the slide in a smaller font size.

    - ○ List complete references for cited materials at the end of the presentation.

- [ ] Use a font size larger than 24 for the slide content and make slide titles slightly larger; references may be in a font that is size 16.

- [ ] Check for consistency in content and formatting.

- [ ] Consider using slide notes as a tool to list additional content to review and cover during an oral presentation.

- [ ] Conclude with implications for practice, research, policy, and future directions.

- [ ] Practice presenting the content for completeness, timing, and flow. Add slides to transition content, if needed.

- [ ] Proofread. Check spelling. Edit. Repeat.

- [ ] Save it! Back it up!
- [ ] Submit the presentation according to specifications but always take a backup copy on a flash drive when you present.
- [ ] Consider whether to have handouts or presentation copies available and submit them ahead of time, if applicable.
- [ ] Allow time for questions.

CITATIONS

American Nurses Association, 2009; Fineout-Overholt, Gallagher-Ford, Mazurek Melnyk, & Stillwell, 2011; Hanrahan, Marlow, Aldrich, & Hiatt, 2012

Tool 12.5   Planning for an EBP Publication

INSTRUCTIONS: Read author guidelines carefully. Review and discuss the checklist as a team:

- ☐ Determine the target audience.
- ☐ Determine authors to invite to participate in writing (be inclusive). Include clinicians on the team.
- ☐ Determine a primary and secondary choice of journals.
- ☐ Read several issues of potential journals if you are not familiar with the typical content.
- ☐ Send query letters via email, with or without an abstract, to the editor to determine interest in a full manuscript.
- ☐ Read and follow author guidelines closely.
- ☐ Consider SQUIRE 2.0 guidelines.
- ☐ Outline content.
- ☐ Begin writing by capturing ideas and editing later.
- ☐ Plan to rewrite, rewrite, rewrite.
- ☐ Use American Psychological Association (APA) formatting until editing is complete, to avoid confusion with numbering citations during review and edits.
- ☐ Complete final content edits before doing final formatting.
- ☐ Include an acknowledgement of funding sources and individuals providing assistance.
- ☐ Review author guidelines again, prior to submission.
- ☐ After submission, consider reviewers' suggestions carefully and be prepared to edit or address their suggestions.
- ☐ If the manuscript is not accepted, consider resubmitting to another journal.

CITATIONS

Adams, Farrington, & Cullen, 2012; American Nurses Association, 2009; Fineout-Overholt, Gallagher-Ford, Mazurek Melnyk, & Stillwell, 2011; Hanrahan, Marlow, Aldrich, & Hiatt, 2012; Holland & Watson, 2012; Roush, 2017a, 2017b; Saver, 2014